Fiona,

Many Blessings to you my Soul Sister.

You have been a great source of Comfort & Love on my Journey. I LOVE YOU!

Peggy (Margaret) Brigham

The wisdom of the Goddess has come to remind us to embrace the "play", in playing golf! I am grateful for this book in that it brings a fresh new outlook to this wonderful game, one that respects Mother Nature and our true nature. May this be a guide to your evolution as a player and a human being.

Jody Jackson,
Class A, LPGA Teaching Professional

"This book takes women on a journey into the self, the body, the mind, the spirit and connects it with the game of golf and the game of life. If you are looking to massively improve your golf game and life game you must read this book."

-Bob Burnham
Author of the # 1 Amazon Best Seller:
101 Reasons Why You Must Write A Book;
How To Make A Six Figure Income By Writing & Publishing Your Own Book

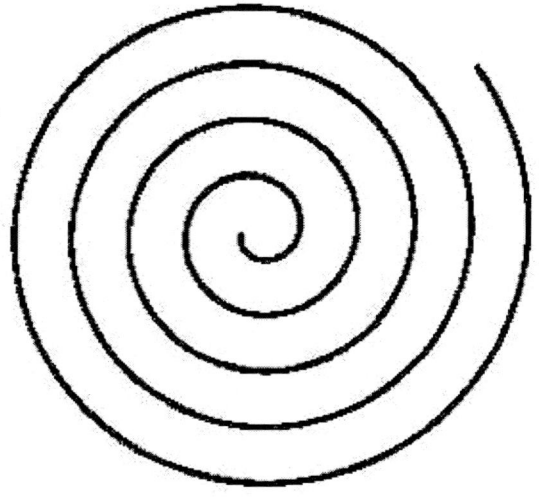

Cover Design- Jim Brigham
Photography by Dave Lund and Paulo Andrade

Copyright © 2008 by Margarit Brigham
All Rights Reserved.

http://www.golfinggoddesses.com

Unauthorized duplication or distribution is strictly prohibited.

ISBN 10: 1-933817-50-X
ISBN 13: 978-1933817-50-7

First Printing: December 2008

Publishing in the USA by
Profits Publishing of Blaine, Washington

http://ProfitsPublishing.com

**Dedicated:
To all my Relatations**

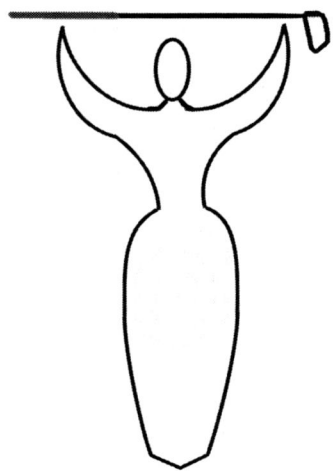

A Yoga for Golf and Goddess Yoga Testimonial:

"Being relatively new to the game of golf (a novice actually), I did not realize how much was involved in learning and playing the game and the level of commitment that is required. For most everyone, the obvious is learning and trying to the master the techniques. However, there is another side to the game that I think a great deal of people overlook. And that is learning how to control your mind and thoughts throughout your game. I had heard and read that this is a significant component to playing successfully.

However, it is not something that I have come across in any book or magazine and it is not something that the average golf instructor incorporates into their teaching. When I was asked by a colleague if I was interested in participating in a yoga for golf program, I did not hesitate to join because I thought that it would help improve my flexibility as it related to the game. What I did not realize was that the yoga for golf program also focused on the mental aspects of the game.

With each class, Margarit gave us a foundation in which we could build on. We learned how to best use our minds in the game. Something that the books and magazines say you should do, but don't tell you how. The breathing techniques to calm your body helped to focus on the shot ahead. The physical stretching and poses help with the flexibility.

Both of these techniques, generally, are also a great way to unwind and release the days' tensions. As for the mental aspect, the visualization is a great tool. If you can visualize where your next shot will go, there is a greater chance that that is where it will land. The power of positive thinking is very key in this game and I think Margarit really shows you how to achieve this. I would recommend the program to others. The techniques that Margarit gives you can be easily incorporated in your everyday practice. It can make a difference in your game."

- Kelly Boreham of North Vancouver B.C.

Goddess Yoga-

*"I wish to share my experience attending, Margarit's Goddess Yoga Class.
I found it captivating, a very powerful journey.
It allowed and taught me how to connect with universal energy in a
very feminine and profound way.
It gave me great tools and insight to use in my everyday life, which
expanded my way of thinking and seeing things in a more divine light.
It allowed me to express myself fully, through yoga and dance, with
much compassion and a greatness of self worth, and creativity.
It showed me how to honor this amazing essence of myself, which was
truly a wonderful gift, and a magical experience.
I wish to give Margarit great thanks for sharing her gifts with me.
They will remain with me always - I feel truly blessed."*

Namaste,
- Goddess Sharon McArthur

Acknowledgments

At times our own light goes out and is rekindled by a spark from an other person. Each of us has cause to think with deep gratitude of those who have lighted the flame within us.
--Albert Schweitzer

I feel blessed to have found the Goddess and the loving relationship I have developed with her over the years. It has been an amazing journey to have the guidance in my life and the inspiration for many words on these pages. I am so grateful for the many gifts on this journey of becoming and I am still in awe many times of the unending love, support and messages that comes from within and in the external events she has brought me to along my path.

I am forever grateful to all the teachers I have studied with, especially Elder Dave Courchene Jr. who helped wake me up to the magic of connecting with everything in the natural world. As well as all the spiritual people that have walked just ahead of me, whether I studied with them in person or in their books, all the gathered knowledge has helped shape my life and life of this book.

I am deeply indebted to all the people I have taught and I am so glad our paths have crossed, the similarities between my students and my friends are; some are in my life a short time, some stay longer and some leave and come back. Sharon and Stu McArthur, and Fiona Wright have been the most magical connection with coming in and out of my life, although I know every connection is special, regardless if they are my family, friends or students. I am grateful to the countless women I have been in ceremony with over the years. In full moon circles, full moon sweat lodges, changing of the seasons and meditation groups, too many women to mention but I hold you all in my heart and healing meditations.

The most loving appreciation goes to my wonderful children; Kim and Daniel, who have not always understood their mom, but still have been a great source of support and selflessness, while I walked this path. A Big Thanks goes to my brothers for their generosity, patience love and support. I am also thankful for all the support from my extended family over the years and to connecting with the Winnipeg clan since our drive out west and my Aunt Betty for supporting the first draft of this book and taking time to edit it

A huge heartfelt THANK YOU to my loving, supportive, life partner Paulo, who helped me tremendously while writing this book, he is very in tune with the Goddess energy and our countless conversations have helped me with clarity and grounded ness many times while writing.

I am deeply grateful to my book mentor Bob Burnham and Jodi Bepler the editor of Profits Publishing for her ongoing assistance, patience and so much time and energy to help bring this book to print.

A Special thank you to the Lady Golf Pro's that have supported my Yoga for Golf business, in the early years it was Shelley Woolner in Ontario, now in B.C. it has been Jeri O'hara and Jody Jackson.

Finally I thank the spirits of my parents Carolyn and Norm Brigham, who I continue to feel close to. I have discovered I can still call upon them anytime for advice and I do receive their messages back in the form of signs and symbols.

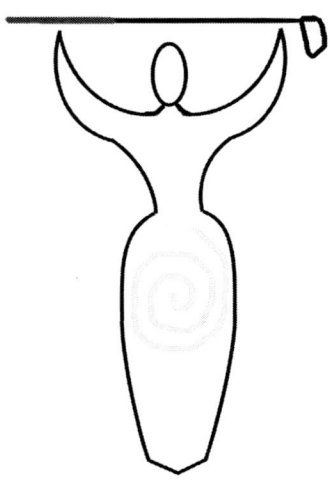

Recipe for Golfing Goddesses

- Say YES to the rhythm of life, Yes to the rhythm of Golf
- Stretch, get to know your body
- Breathe slowly to live longer
- Repeat affirmations frequently
- Set goals and visualize them already complete
- Be radical, break away from conscious mind thinking to the sub-conscious mind doing.
- Play in a sacred way, in union with mother earth and nature
- Be still, be silent
- Listen to your body and your intuition
- Believe in something, know what your spiritual beliefs are and incorporate them into your day
- Simplify
- Become healthier as you age, every moment that passes is an opportunity for change
- Live in the moment, right here.
- Take frequent negativity diets from the news, sources like Radio, T.V. Newspapers, and even People
- Dare, "Fate loves the Fearless"
- See the Glass half full
- Raise your vibration, play gratitude games
- Develop your imagination to become child-like
- Remember that it is never too late to begin

"The game of golf is like the game of life...the goal is to develop to your highest potential and become self-governing!"

–Margarit Brigham

Table of Contents

Why Become a Golf Goddess? 13
The Authors quest in Becoming 16
How to Become a Golf Goddess? 23
Symbolism of the Circle 30

Part 1 – Direction East- Element Air 32

Chapter 1 *Oya* - African Goddess 33
Hole 1   - Transformation 34
Hole 10 – Confidence 44

Chapter 2 *Isis* Egyptian Goddess 53
Hole 2   - Pranayama/Yogic Breathing 54
Hole 11 – Relaxation 65

Part 2 - Direction South - Element Fire 70

Chapter 3 *Pele* - Hawaiian Goddess 71
Hole 3 - Passion 73
Hole12 – Freedom 80

Chapter 4 *Kali* - Hindu Goddess 84
Hole 4   - Patience 85
Hole 13 – Persistence 90

Part 3 – Direction West- Element Water 94

Chapter 5 *Coventina* - Scottish Goddess 95
Hole 5   - Balance 96
Hole 14 – Flexibility 99

Chapter 6 *Sedna* - Inuit Goddess 103
Hole 6   - Intuition 105
Hole 15 – Focus..112

Part 4– Direction North- Element Earth .. 116

Chapter 7   *Gaia* - Greek Goddess 117
Hole 7   - Mother Earth 118
Hole 16 - Sacred Play 133

Chapter 8 *Artemis* -Greek Goddess 140
Hole 8   - Grounding...142
Hole 17 – Intention 150

Part 5 –Direction Center-Element Ether .. 154

Chapter 9 *Tara* -Tibetan Goddess 155
Hole 9   - Centering 156
Hole 18 - The Zone...163

Sacred Golf Journeys: A New Dawn 173
Yoga Introduction and Warm-ups......................................179
Yoga Poses...182
Targeted Golf Areas 197
Bibliography 200
Resources: Books 201
Resources: Other 202
Authors Biography 203

Introduction

Why Become A Golf Goddess?

"Why the Goddesses? Because we are women, diverse women, who need to see the Divine Feminine, reflected back to us - from ourselves to our Goddesses and back to ourselves. Because all women are Goddesses, and it is time we saw ourselves that way!!"

Excerpts from *"The Goddess Oracle"*
by Amy Sophia Marashinsky

What does it mean to be a golf goddess compared to just being a woman golfer? Becoming a golf goddess is playing in closer relationship to who we are as females and to reconnect back to our own natural rhythms. Golf is a perfect playing field to discover and uncover who we really are as a female species and how much we have been hurting since we have been disconnected with our own natural flow. Each of us has a unique path that is right for us; one of the quickest ways to find it is by being in a relationship to Mother Earth and the feminine Energy. Golfers have a unique opportunity to fast track this relationship since we can be outside playing for hours. Play being the operative word here. The Goddesses are calling to us all, and women have been hearing the call the most. Our Mother needs our attention and Love and that is a very simple act we can all perform. Since we are multidimensional we will find certain Goddesses resonate with us at different times. The more attention we pay to certain goddesses the more that energy type comes back to offer us guidance. When we see evidence of help from the higher realms, a spontaneous appreciation occurs. This then becomes a wonderful cyclical flow of asking, receiving and being grateful. The more frequently we are outside, the more we can receive messages, information and intuition from nature. The purpose of this book is to bring women a step closer towards sacredness and play on the golf courses and then it will spill over into every area of our lives effortlessly. I Live a life Extraordinaire since becoming a Golf Goddess and I truly desire the same for you!

On your way to becoming you will discover you are actually co-creating your games and your lives with a more wise and loving energy, which I happen to call the Goddess of Golf. Over the years she has introduced herself to me with many symbols and signs that are like a lighthouse when I am in the fog about what path to take and when to take it. When you get to know her in your life, you will see she encompasses a much bigger territory then just the golf courses.

One day your focal point will change and you will begin to look at your playing golf as a journey, a path to the Heart and to the Hero within. In other words a journey back to unconditional Love. You will find even if you are not playing you are always a player of the game and you will observe how your life lessons can be learned whether you are on the golf course or not. When viewed rightly, your lifestyle becomes a game. When you play at life you attract more good things as you are living at higher vibrations. All men and women have an intuitive intelligence and this book is about waking that up, bringing it out and playing it out.

The first thing to become comfortable with is learning how Nature communicates with her children, the language of Nature speaks in the form of symbols.

We all come from nature, we are all connected to the natural world, but we have lost the ability to understand the messages and how to live in harmony. The wonderful thing about the age of technology is we don't have to look far to begin the search. Because of the internet all we need is at our fingertips, we need only apply discernment and a trial and error process to find what works best for us. You will find some of the language of nature in this book, others I leave for you to discover on your own. Never worry, there isn't any right or wrong way to search or to live, for example, the spiritual people I know have been truth seekers for many years; they have studied many different paths and healing modalities. Everyone has a story about why they started searching and even though they have gone different ways to find the truth for them, we can all understand each other, even if the words used are a bit different. So their lives reflect and include bits and pieces from many sources. It would be difficult to say anyone one of them lives just one way now, as a religious person, as a Buddhist, as a Zen, as a pagan. No, today's people are more complex and encompassing then the people of yesterday's, who seemed content as a whole to stay on one path or religious doctrine, because that is what they were born into.

Today we are very fortunate, we have more freedom, and we can begin to play golf as a spiritual experience, which will heal and shape our lives. We can begin to move through golf, business and life using the Laws of Nature or, "Universal Laws" which are more life affirming and are in-fused with love, in comparison to man-made laws that cause separation. As we come back to our true selves we begin to heal and change the planet. The Goddess tradition embraces play and pleasure, all acts of love and pleasure were seen as a ritual to her, a way to honor and praise her. The more we honor and celebrate this life; the more grace descends down on us.

I once read that both the Koran, the sacred book of Islam and the Talmud the

Come, Be Golfing Goddesses!

sacred book of the Jewish; teach- "that we will be called to account for every permissible pleasure life offered us, but which we refused to enjoy while on earth?"

It's time my sisters, to begin to play everyday, in everyway. As a buy product of becoming a Golf Goddess you can participate fully in paving the way for a new balanced world. Think about what we are passing on now, whether you have children or not, whether you are a child starting golf right now or a grandmother, most peoples lives are lived in habits, many habits of fear and distrust have been fed to us. We pass up permissible pleasure all the time; we have been conditioned to be a dead society. The life of our inner core is just waiting for us to turn towards it. What will you find? The wonder and magic that weaves itself through all of life, now flowing through yours. Welcome to the adventure!

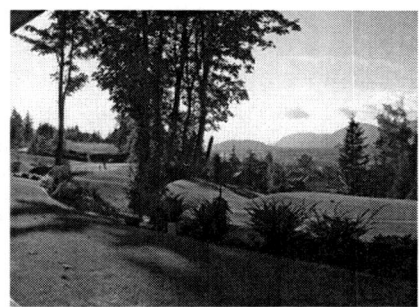

My Journey in Becoming

"One vision I see clear as life before me, is that the ancient mother has awakened once more, sitting on her throne rejuvenated, more glorious then ever. Proclaim her to the entire world with the voice of peace and benediction".

- Vivekananda

This journey to combine yoga with golf was inspired when I started working at golf courses in the early 1990's. I had been a bartender for years and I was drained from listening to the customer's problems. I decided I wanted to work at a place where people were happy. I thought golf clubs would be a good place to work because people were there to play a game. Boy was I wrong. I find out many golfers were as stressed out and miserable as my old customers and I couldn't understand it. I used to think, "Hey, they were not at work and they were playing in natural beautiful surroundings what's the problem?" The first golf course I worked at was considered a championship course, I got to play for free and I was a beginner, I had played a bit with my parents growing up but not on golf courses such as Lionhead in Ontario. Boy, did I learn how the game could become frustrating, not the best for beginners. By the time I went to work at another golf course I was taking my yoga teacher training and I immediately saw how easily yoga transferred to the game. The mind/body connection is a fantastic transformational tool for better golf and here was a solution to help golfers become happier.

This is how it worked for me; before I went out to play I would do yoga in the ladies locker. At that time in 1994 I didn't notice anyone else stretching before games or stretching at the driving range and I used to get all kinds of funny looks. I didn't care when I played at the course I worked at, but it made me feel too intimidated when I played golf at any other courses. So I wouldn't warm up ("I was not very evolved at the time and now it doesn't matter who is watching I have inner confidence and belief, I know what is best for me and I will follow that rather than be intimidated by other peoples thoughts, opinions and beliefs.")

In those early days I discovered if I didn't warm up it would take until the fourth hole to be performing at my best. Alternatively when I stretched and warmed up I was performing my best on the first tee. I also became aware that stretching before hand relieved my first tee jitters. Then came the day after my second year into my Teacher Training program I realized how wonderful the yoga principles for the mind and emotions were for playing golf. Having this discipline, I learned was even more significant than having all my shots perfected, to play an enjoyable game.

The concepts I was learning in my yoga class like being in the moment, non-attachment, positive attitude, going with the flow, tolerance, discipline, acceptance, honesty and humility were such great tools to have when playing golf. My whole game transformed. I realized the yoga concepts became deeper ingrained while I played, because golf brings instant results. The golf course honestly shows you, where your state of mind is. (Is it a battlefield, or is it a playground)? When I realized the golf course was a battlefield for most golfers I became saddened. More than anything, I knew the concepts I was learning could help golfers become more relaxed and happy. So I was inspired to become an entrepreneur and begin a business which I simply named Yoga for Golf my mission was to bring happiness to golfers. I was a pioneer trying to bring a new concept into the golf industry and it was a hard sell, it wasn't until 1997 that I finally taught my first session at a golf course and they only wanted the fitness aspect of yoga. My quest to help golfers become happier began to shape my own life as well as help me to teach the happiness skills in all my yoga classes, general yoga or otherwise. I learned to become my own best friend and to coach others to believe in themselves. A lot of my confidence came through my own trial and error and I had to walk many parts of the journey alone for awhile. I have had to walk my talk not only in golf, but also through my personal and business life. For so many years I was my own encouragement. My ideas were not supported by many golfers; oh they thought the ideas were unique however the fear of trying something new was a big deterrent for them to try it for themselves.

Then one fine summer day, many years later, I went golfing with three friends. One of them would refer to me as a golfing goddess throughout the game. It stuck with me because it made me feel empowered. Since then, I now use this phrase while golfing with other women. The fun part is watching the change that occurs on the golf course. First a sparkle comes to their eyes and a shy smile forms when I first call them a Golf Goddess. By the end of the day their smile is wider, eyes are more sparkling, and their stride is more confident. I can clearly see the goddess emerge in their body language. I'm not sure how conscious the other person is, but some part of her sure remembers. It is my deepest wish to bring forth the Goddess energy for all females, to reawaken, and reclaim our power as women and golfers.

It is not only my goal; you see I have been commissioned to write this by The Universe/The Goddess. The name of the book and the outline came when I was very ill. At that time I did not begin writing in earnest, I was too busy being a single parent while simultaneously expanding myself as a businesswoman by opening and operating my own yoga studio, The Yoga Connection in a small town of Orangeville Ontario. Things were running along fine for quite a few years, but then the bottom of my world dropped out when I lost both of my parents within three and one-half weeks of each other.

My parents' death became the beginning of a deep letting go of a number of aspects in my life. Many changes occurred in a very short time from releasing my Yoga studio, my home, friends, most of my material possessions. Leaving my grown children and buying a little trailer and driving out to B.C., apparently all for the birth of this book. The writing of this book has helped many pieces of the puzzles make sense and what my life's purpose is. I realize a few things about the timing of when the book had to be written, seven years after I received the vision. I now know, I had to be empty enough to become a channel for the ideas to come through me and I had to go through more ceremony with my partner, who has in turn been a huge process to this book.

In the two years of writing we have had many conversations that have sparked parts of the book. It was truly a partnership effort; he was open enough to be a channel for the Goddess energy to speak through him to me. Ladies, I must go off track for a moment and tell you all the principles in this book, will not only help you create great golf, but any aspect in your life. i.e.: Attracting your soul mate. The laws of attraction do work to bring a relationship if that is what you desire in an easy and relaxed way. Believe me; I did not think I could let love in my life after the pain of losing my parents. It seemed too much a risk to open my heart and enter a relationship, only to go though more heartache, no way. Then I was told in a psychic reading, a man was on the way, I had mixed feelings I wanted one, but I was too scared. So I did a ceremony in a special place, I left a gift for mother earth and I wrote a list of what I wanted in a partner, then I let the whole process go and went on with my healing which was my biggest priority. I knew what I didn't want.

I was in a long term common-law and then marriage of a total of 17 years and then a few relationships which all helped me grow to some extent. But where I really learned to love myself was by being single, and relying on myself through two big major events, when I opened my yoga studio and going through the year of taking care of my parents and then through the loss of both of them in such a short time.

I had the comfort and strength of my higher Self who would bring the right support in the form of friends, books, music and even movies. It was a process in which I learned to balance my inner male and inner female and without looking I found a supportive partner on the outside who I was later told was also going through the same process of learning about his inner male and female.

Throughout this book you will discover different ways I reveal the secrets to manifesting. Everything must first begin with the inner work before it shows up on the outside. Over the years I learned to follow my inner Goddess; my intuition by trail and error, especially in my professional life. Along the way my life and my life's work became one. The Yoga Teacher Training course was transformational for my spiritual life and I couldn't get enough. In those early years I was forever researching the new concepts I had learned about, by continuing to study, going to workshops and seminars, mainly through the Learning Annex. One of my yoga teachers was my inspiration for researching the Goddess. My awakening to the Goddess energy or, as one of my friends told me, my "initiation", came before I started my Yoga for Golf business, but I didn't do much with it at the time except journal about it. I have been journaling for years, journaling my adventures into the spiritual life, my dreams and visions and especially my life's challenges and struggles.

Looking back in my journals, I have recorded in 1995, the experience of this awakening. I was meditating after a day-long workshop with Wayne Dyer and I fell asleep and became conscious of a voice in my mind, which said to me, "Everyone loves God but no one loves Mary". From some place inside myself, another voice of mine answered, "I will". Then a wave of Love so strong came over me, it had me sitting bolt upright and gasping for breath I was so scared, it took my breath away. Actually I was terrified and couldn't go back to sleep. I was still with my ex-husband and he slept through the whole thing, which I found unbelievable because it seemed like a lighting bolt came right through the room. But the experience didn't end that night, over the next couple of months, just out of the blue; people would start sharing experiences they had with Mary. For example they would say they read a book on Mother Mary and would lend it to me, this happened a couple of times and it wasn't always friends who knew me or about my experience.

I have since learned Mother Mary can be interpreted into the Goddess, Queen of Heaven, like Inanna before her, but being raised Catholic I am interpreting Spirit's message to me that the feminine form had to be one I could associate with at the time. As I started my research about Mary I also saw her as Isis; how she was here well before Christianity gave her the name Mary. I didn't do anything with this experience until a couple of years later when I wanted to give up on Yoga for Golf. I was getting quite discouraged by all the rejection of this unique program, it was only seasonal and I could only get a few classes going at best in the early days.

I remembered some part of me said "I would love the Goddess (Mary)" and so I created a Goddess Yoga program as a way to honor her. I hoped I would learn more about the Goddess by others who came and took the class. My teacher used to say, "We teach what we most need to learn." And I needed to learn about this energy before I could love it. The classes were the most fun and creative sessions I ever taught, but the Yoga for Golf kept persisting. Signs and coincidences kept occurring until I surrendered, quite loudly I might add, I had a temper tantrum with the Universe; with my energy spent I became humbled. I truly surrendered, I had the awareness that Yoga for Golf was part of my life's work, my Dharma and I needed to learn as much from this path as I needed to teach it. Through the years

I had the trust, patience and perseverance to stick with the path. Now I am doing what I truly love, what I am passionate about connecting women back to the land in a sacred way through a game.

Although most of this book to help women find a spiritual path and their inner core by playing the game of golf is based on the teachings from my Yoga for Golf classes. I also draw from my studies and experiences from the Native Path and learning about the goddesses and other earth based traditions which helped me create Goddess Yoga.

I use these examples through-out, to help us understand the Laws of Nature, because connecting to the inner core is really about living a life connected to the path of the heart and this path is in many cultures. Similarly as the Goddess was revered in many countries; she encompassed many aspects. I have been fortunate enough to attract many teachers both men and women who are in harmony with the lessons taught by nature and the earth. They may not use the word Goddess but the energy is still the same. I feel confident that all my sisters upon this planet can easily relate with the Goddess because she has many faces in every race. The many faces of the Goddess are all, the one Goddess.

Just like the moon has many phases it is still one moon. You will find throughout the book the Goddesses of the East, West, North and South which all come together to create a balance. My Yoga for Golf logo is a Yin and Yang. I have always used balance in my teaching of the body for golfers but also in the holistic aspect of teaching the whole person not just the body. The balance between all parts of a person the spirit, mind, body, and emotions or heart, empowers golfers with the knowledge of how to create great golf. I have been shown that by learning to trust and depend on my intuitive intelligence I can create golf games and life games with excitement, power and natural magical moments over and over again. Writing this book has brought me more awareness on how I can help point the way through my own examples and others I have taught to bring these same aspects to anyone's life. A wholeness or synergy has emerged where I do not have separate compartments for my life, my work, my relationship or my play. By becoming a Golfing Goddess myself, it has dawned on me that I have been walking the path of the heart without truly noticing it until I wrote this book.

The light has been shed, but I have been put through many tests of courage and risks before I could even get to the stage to begin writing. With awareness we can see that even though society wants us to live by the liner ticking clock that is only an illusion. Nature shows us that the true way to live life and all its many aspects lies within a circular form. This book is intentionally laid out in a circular format; although it seems circular events have written their way into the lay out since it has been a two year process of writing.

Writing this book has been a process of patience since many times I believed it to be finished because I wanted to be in control. I have had to surrender control of the timing over and over again. When I let this be what it really is a co-creative effort with the Goddess I reconnect to the Universes flow or The Way. When I finally became serious and started writing this book to the exclusion of being driven by outside influences like, time, money, and big responsibilities, everything showed up at the right time. I have used the term Law of Attraction, many times throughout the book because it is a term that people are familiar with. Although what I have been really following is the ancient way called the Tao.

The Law of least resistance, or the Taoist principle termed another way Wu Wei Wu which teaches 'do without doing' and everything gets done.' I was doing, by writing this book, the evidence of without doing, came in the form of support from my partner, then later from mentors, learning about publishing, and finally about marketing, all came to me as outer resources, as I was internally asking for the next step to reveal itself.

The final transformation for this book came in 2008 was volunteering as messenger, fundraiser and event co-coordinator for my favorite charity, Turtle Lodge in Manitoba. My teacher Native Elder Dave Courchene built it for all races, a place to come and learn. Then a woman did a documentary on him and a Native Prophecy called the 8th Fire. I brought what is termed the 8th Fire Experience to B.C., which involves a screening of the movie and Dave's presence to give a personal talk because to see him in a movie is not as powerful as seeing him live since he is a pure channel for spirits message. And his message is very important for humanity at this time as we move closer to the year 2012. In this book you will be introduced to him from my experiences of being in ceremony with him and by passing on his teachings that I have recorded over the 13 years I have known him.

Since my involvement in bringing his message forth I have noticed my writing has changed and is more influenced by the Mother Earth herself. I feel as if she is using me as a bridge between the unconventional thinkers and the conventional ones, to help close the gap of separation that we may all join together on the same playing field. I offer hope to inspire my female spiritual friends and my family who will be reading this book, and are not golfers, to join this path of becoming Golfing Goddesses and help shift the way to oneness and harmony not only our human family but with the natural world as well.

Finally I would like to share another aspect on my way to Becoming a Golf Goddess, my name has been transformed. My given name is Margaret and most Scottish people know that Margaret has many nicknames, Peggy being one of them. I was called Peggy growing up, and I had a heck of a time when dealing with legal documents explaining I was both Margaret and Peggy. With the decision to move to a new Province I decided that I would use my given name Margaret since I would be getting a new drivers license, health card, etc. Although, through a series of events, I have given myself a new nickname in 2006, more of a Goddess name which is Margarit pronounced Margaruitte. Now I have become a proud Grandmother - yes, we are always still becoming.

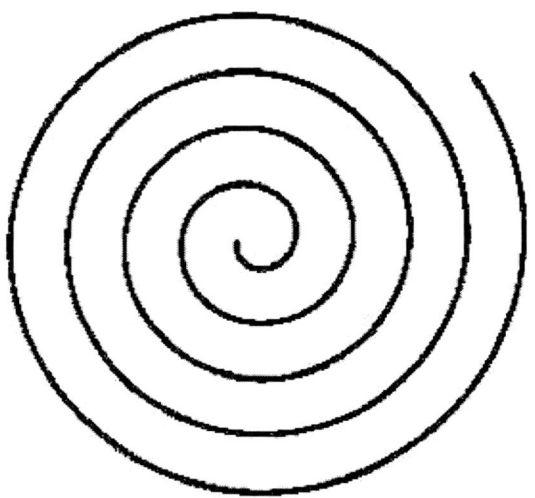

Foundation

How to Become Golf Goddess?

"Golf is a game of virtues, but these virtues can remain in the seed state. Adding the discipline of yoga is like adding rays of sunshine it helps to illuminate the virtues. Our life path can then be viewed as a seed. With the right conditions we do not stay in the limiting confines of the shell. We break free of the incased shell, push up through dirt, get rained on and buffeted by wind, until one day we blossom and even have the potential to bear fruit."

-MB

To Grow or not to Grow? *"Growing is the most important and essential endeavor that a human being can undertake. You can make and lose money; you can be promoted and demoted in the world. Never, at any stage, is there any certainty about what will happen to you in this life. However, there is one thing that nobody can ever take away from you-the growth you attain through your own search for Self-knowledge. Furthermore, this growth and understanding become the foundation that sustains you through any and all worldly difficulties, and that allow you- whatever the form of your physical experience-to find in life a continuously unbroken flow of total well-being."*

-Swami Chetanananda

From a yogic standpoint many Guru's would have their disciples begin to work on their inner discipline and higher moral qualities before introducing the Yoga poses (asanas) and breathing techniques (pranayama). I feel that golf has helped prepare us along this route, since inherent within the game is not only the golf etiquette, which develops courtesy and respect for the golf course and other players, but also the higher morals that can be learned from playing. When viewed in its truest form, golf is a game that teaches virtues such as honesty, integrity, patience, and humility to name but a few. All golfers may get these lessons but many do not embrace them as treasures to build, more often then not they are a constant source of frustration. Over the years golf industry has done a great job of masking the inner game and draws the focus on the outer. Developing the best balls, clubs, shoes, and clothes, are all fine but have little significance to Golfing Goddesses.

Although as in the game of life, there have been signposts along the way if we are searching into the mysteries in golf, a great book *'Golf in the Kingdom'* helped open the ones who were ready. The masses were not at the time but hang on ladies because we are raising our energies more as a group consciousness and all the spiritual golf books that have been published before their time will be very useful to help keep this new way of seeing and being alive.

We begin the journey by inquiring into the truth of the words, play natures way, naturally. The biggest disservice the golf industry has done is by making the learning of swinging a golf club very unnatural. Sure it has succeeded as a big money maker, getting everyone to buy into the idea that they need lessons over and over again. This is madness, and it is not improving a golfer's game at all. It has frustrated and drained golfers of confidence, passion, money and time. Why does this happen? Because the traditional way of teaching has been very unbalanced, focusing over and over on the mechanics, by this I mean the endless pointers and tips are for the mind and the thinking conscious brain. This is not helpful and the results are in, golfers are not improving over the past years even though the equipment keeps on improving. The natural way to learn something new is a two step process-

Natural Learning Process

1. When learning something new it begins with commands to the body, and that happens by the use of conscious mind. When first learning, our movements look sloppy, erratic at first. This is because there are many different instructions to focus on all at once.

2. Then the next step, information gets stored in the body and subconscious mind. This results in an effortless, smooth functioning of automatic pilot response.

For example, riding a bicycle as humans we don't need to learn to ride a bike every few years. No, once it is integrated, once our bodies are taught to do this we don't ever have to think about it consciously again. If we did we would continuously look erratic in our performance. I use an example of driving a standard car further in the book.

Can you see the natural two step way of learning with anything, learning a musical instrument, learning to skate, and ski? Luckily learning to swing a baseball bat or tennis racket is not taught like learning to swing a golf club. For me this is the masculine way of learning, from the liner, logical side. As I mentioned this way is unbalanced, to correct the situation I will be introducing the feminine way of learning in this book. Learning to allow each moment to happen naturally, to be soft in body, to use more creative visualization these qualities and more that you will read about will help correct years of being taught only the swing mechanics as the way to play better golf.

Now the LPGA is becoming much more balanced in teaching new ways to learn Golf; compared to only techniques and mechanics. But when it comes right down to it, trying to be in control, is an insult. Humans are such powerful beings and have miraculous bodies, imagine trying to give instructions on making the heart pump, the digestive system to eliminate and all the other countless functions the subconscious does on its own. We have been taught and conditioned in an unnatural way, a one step process. This means as golfers we have our work cut out for us, to unlearn the unnatural teaching methods. You may say "oh I understand now the two-step process way of learning, I got it!" and I can stop reading now.

People are constantly surprised when they think they understand a new concept and then try to integrate it without replacing the bad habits with the new ones. Don't underestimate the forms of resistance that will arise, this long held belief is so ingrained that it will take work to switch back to the natural way. Sounds crazy I know, but we are creatures of habit and you will encounter blocks from within and without. However, I know from experience that the little bit of work on building proper habits yields wonderful results I have found it is worth it. You will discover so many benefits by encompassing this balanced approach to your learning and playing.

What you have to understand is this book is all about the application of breaking down years of habits so you can begin your own journey of become golfing goddesses. We do this through learning to play more in the vibration of feminine energy. Since we play outside upon Mother Earth the wisdom of playing nature's way can come easily. I will be describing what the Feminine way of Golf really means throughout the book. One way I do this is by incorporating many earth based traditions that live or lived closer to the earth and the seasons which is a more in tune with the feminine way. In this book I will not be giving a history lesson of the Goddess tradition. I will be explaining how the energies of the different goddesses I picked for golf can be played out in our lives. I will draw upon their archetypes and myth, although using my own slant on each goddess and how she can be related to the game of golf.

Let's look at the similarity to draw upon between Golf and the Goddess way of living, Goddess teachings are circular i.e.: following the seasons, as opposed to a liner, straight line of progressive thinking. If we look at the way golf courses are laid out they also form a circle, you begin at the clubhouse and then end at the clubhouse. The holes do not go in a straight line. How boring would that be? Any female can use the principles in this book whether she is a youth (a princess), an adult (a Queen) or a grandmother (a wise woman) all will benefit. You will notice along the way to becoming a Golfing Goddess yourself that you will begin to walk the path of the heart and gain more powerful drives, and powerful lives.

At this point I would like to explain the different yoga traditions used in this book and how they differ from most of the western world's knowledge on Yoga. Many people think of yoga in terms of a fitness program that is only one path and it is called Hatha yoga. I have combined Hatha yoga, Raja yoga and the devotional path called Bhakti Yoga into the make up of a Golfing Goddesses program. Now, Raja yoga is referred to as "The Royal Road" which has more to do with the mind. It is the highest path of yoga there is.

There are many paths to yoga, the word yoga translated means union or joining together. The way my yoga teacher explained it is by using a metaphor of climbing a mountain. She told us "India is a country that's spiritual beliefs are more important then material, the main emphasis is on reaching samahdi this word can be likened to enlightenment. The ancient yogis were forest dwellers and they learned about the human being while studying the mind through meditation, the body through observing and living in nature and then devised the systems of yoga or a union for our whole selves, inside and out. "The yogis see all humans climbing up the mountain to reach enlightenment, even if some people are not aware of it in this life, the yogis know they will reach the mountain in another life. Through developing an understanding of the human psyche, the yogis determined not all people had the same disposition. So the best and quickest way to the top is to find the yoga path or paths that best suits their temperament."

Besides the three I mentioned there are other paths, and some people inter mix the paths to best suit them. There is also Karma yoga, which is the yoga of selfless action if you ever volunteer you are doing Karma yoga. Jhana yoga, which is learning through spiritual scripture, it is more suited for the intellectual nature. Bhakti yoga, which is Hindu's most popular discipline, is more emotional and includes mantras and devotion to the Divine, in whatever form the Divine takes for each person. Believe me since I have adopt this attitude to be tolerant and accepting of all peoples choices on the form of worship they wish to devote their lives to, it has been so freeing.

The three main yoga paths for Golfing Goddesses are Hatha Yoga, Raja Yoga and Bhakti Yoga below is a brief introduction to them:

Hatha Yoga -Yoga is an ancient form of self-improvement, with scientifically proven results. In general yoga stretches move at a slower pace than other forms of fitness, giving discipline and focus two essential components required in golf. Practiced daily, yoga for golf stretches relieve tension and stress, helps reclaim lost energy and improve overall sports performance.

Raja Yoga Philosophy - One important point that I have recently begun to share in my workshops and classes is that; Most people over the years have asked the question "what is the meaning of yoga? which most know means a union of the mind, body and spirit. Now we want to ask the next question 'What is Yoga?' This can be answered properly from Pantanjali "Yoga is a control of the thought-waves in your mind." Now who is Pantanjali you may ask? He is known in the yoga world as the Father of Yoga. The way knowledge was passed down was verbally from Guru to disciple. Patanjali was the first to put it down Yoga in a book form over 1500 years ago. The very first Book (which is known as a Pada) is called; Yoga and its Aims

The first sutra is what most of the Western world thinks of yoga but it is the very next sutra that is important to the game of golf.

1. This is the beginning of instruction in yoga – yoga basically means union- hence comes the words Mind/Body/Spirit a yoking, brining the aspirant to wholeness by joining all parts back together.
2. Yoga is a control of thought-waves in the mind. – Releasing the monkey mind chatter so you can hear the inner voice of guidance from your Higher Self.

Patanjali composed a series of sutras, which means *thread*. The sutra was only a sentence or two and then a Master would expand upon the meaning and teaching, threading one sutra to the next.

I like to use the example of a string of pearls for the Goddesses; Pearls of Wisdom. Like the thread in the sutras the pearls are on a string linking one lesson to the next. The lesson of the Pearl is a wonderful one for golf. How does the oyster make a pearl? From a grain of sand. The sand is an irritant and the clam endures the irritation of the grain of sand and eventually is rewarded with a beautiful pearl. So in the manner of life, or the game of golf, we have things that irritate us and, like the oyster, if we are patient and endure we will get rewarded with a beautiful quality of character.

Bhakti Yoga - I would like you to realize that the Goddess has always been worshiped and still is with the Hindu people. She is very much integrated into their lives, as she has never left their scripture. The discipline of devotion, praise and meditation on the inner divine qualities of a Higher Being brings forth the same qualities in us. This is how come Vedic knowledge has been a source of inner peace, profound wisdom, and spiritual inspiration to millions of people since the dawn of time. The Goddess is a symbol of how, when all our good qualities are gathered, they awaken an inner power that destroys negative tendencies. The Goddess represents the potential for all to harness their inner power to overcome negativity and to live in a more joyous existence.

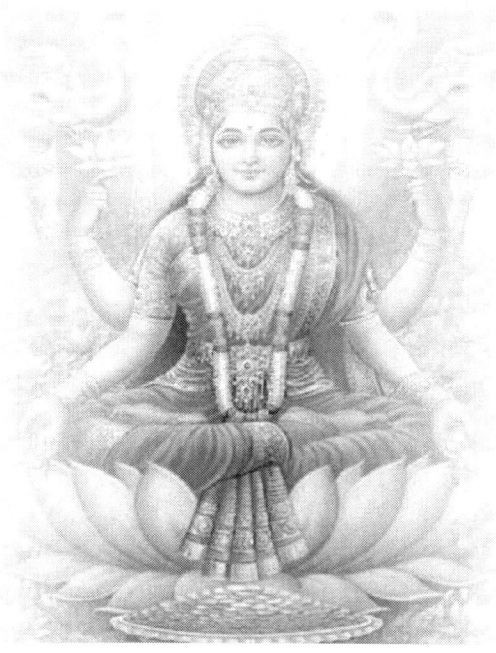

The perfect yoga is not in the outward expression of the poses but a perfect union or integration of our whole beings. How can this knowledge improve your golf game? Think about this… "On the inside the best players are able to clear the mind, concentrate for all 18 holes, overcome frustration, doubt and fear, and develop confidence and patience on every shot."

Nothing else I have tried has given me the above benefits then incorporating both Hatha Yoga and Raja Yoga together.

I have been blessed with a strong imagination and it is this ability to see and try new things that had me creating new and different yoga classes in which I have now combined to make up Golfing Goddesses. This book is written after a decade of teaching and is laid-out in a similar format of two-nine week sessions. In both my Yoga for Golf Classes and Goddess Yoga I have always used themes as a way of sequencing and building one pearl of wisdom to the next. The wonderful outcome is that the teachings within the themes transfer effortlessly from Practice to Play.

To connect to your inner core on a deeper level means to participate with other women in sacred space. We encourage each other to shape shift from a creature crippled with responsibilities and burdened with social expectation into a beautiful wild woman. Anytime I lead Golfing Goddesses classes or a workshop it is in a ceremonial way. Along with you my sisters, we create sacred space and we gain personal power while celebrating women and the Divine at the same time. We allow for this healing space to fully BE, supporting each other that in this space, it is okay to be selfish and look inwards, to let go of the outside world and its wants and needs and to give ourselves permission for this time out. When we come to a class or workshop it is a time for our bonding, for nourishing and caring, that we as women are so good at giving to others. We use the time in Golfing Goddesses workshops to give to each other and ourselves. I have found over the years my sisters yearn for sacred space in which they feel safe to share with their peers. Part of creating the safe space is to support each other and to remember who we are, Spirit in Body.

For the Golfing Goddesses workshops my sisters are encouraged to bring a scarf or sarong to wrap around their yoga clothes for our portion of the warm-up, which is dancing. Dancing is a great way to release trapped energy and raise the vibrational energy to happiness and this energy attracts good things into our lives. The feedback over the years with the Goddess Yoga was the dancing portion was a highlight for everyone. This could be because dancing in sacred space is quite different then going out dancing.

As women we need this connection, I need this, we need others who are supportive, not competitive. We need safe spaces to unwind, to be nurtured, to practice and learn about empowerment. During the last 10 years I have been fortunate to meet many of my sisters in full moon circles, meditation circles, equinox and solstice ceremonies. Not in Wicca circles but with Wicca influences, as well as Native American and now I bring it to the golf circle. I have participated in ceremony in mixed company and through both experiences I have found that there are many more stories that unfold when it is just women connected together.

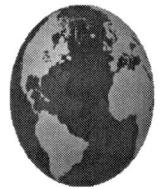 # The Circle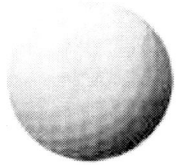

For centuries women of many cultures have met on the half, new, and full moon. In this way they could support each other in deepening their understanding of themselves, others, the Gods, the Goddesses and the cycles of the Earth. Some gathered in temples, ruins, churches, teepees, yurts, tents and others created sacred circles in nature to honor the changing of the seasons with the equinox's, solstices and cross quarter celebrations. When we connect with nature and are truly present with it, we find ourselves again, and recognize the teachings that we are interconnected with all life on this planet.

The circle or orb is an ancient shape that provides human-kind with a sense of completion. It denotes sacred space; it represents cycles – women's cycles, the cycle of life, the cycle of change, the cycle of creativity, the cycle of the golf course. The golf ball is an orb, just like the earth, Venus, Mars and the stars. It is the center of the game.

Women are more tuned into cycles and circular formats. We live by our cycles, we speak in circular formats, and we spiral outward with our energy, and spiral back into our bodies with each monthly cycle. Our bodies are vessels made up of circles. This is why we are so tuned in to emotional cycles, nature's cycle, the cycles of the moon, fire, water and spirit, from which we are inspired to create.

The Golf Course is a cycle. And with its many qualities and challenges it stimulates us to move through it, facing the challenges, learning its course and increasing our skills and abilities. Each challenge is viewed as a teacher; we will never come to an end of the line and say "I've got the lesson" be it patience, persistence, positive thinking. No, we don't travel in a straight line of progress, the lessons come back to be learned at a deeper and deeper level revealing the hero in us.

A Golf Goddess challenges herself on the course. She understands that each hole represents an aspect of the overall cycle she has entered into. Unlike the traditional male model of golf which is linear, competitive and encourages one to "dominate", the female model of golf is circular, co-operative and encouraging one to "grow" and strengthen their power within, not their power over.

We grow into Golfing Goddesses by looking within, by looking at nature with new eyes, by seeing our sisters as mirrors of our feminine self and by using our imaginations. We carry the female vibration and the male vibration inside all of us, the wonderful part is when we are consciously choosing which vibe to bring forth at different times and for different situations, we grow to full maturity. I am asking you to bring forth the female vibe while playing. Look at the successful men who call upon their female vibe to create success in golf. Tiger Woods and Vijah Singh, both have roots in the feminine vibe traditions of Asia and India. Once we can let go of control, the ego & masculine way and be open and willing to 'go with the flow the female vibe, a different rhythm of energy unfolds and guides us, the fun will be in all the adventures along the way.

The lessons of the circle have worked their way into the format of this book using the cycles of nature and the elements also in the way the information has been given to me through my life's experiences while writing this book.

I give you permission to trust your intuition and read this book anyway that feels right to you. If you need a certain topic like patience read that Chapter first. The Centering method in Chapter nine has quickly helped golfer's games so I would recommend reading this Chapter immediately. Be open and willing to try learning in this circular way. This may seem an unfamiliar method of reading but it will help you break free of the progressive straight line conditioning we are trained to live by. Since we are part of nature we do learn and live in a circular way, sometimes we are aware of this, but most times we are not. Approach the book making reading fun by trusting that you will be lead to exactly what you need on a certain day. The right messages will call out to you when you need them. Begin your journey into trusting the Goddess of Golf first while reading this book, then it will be easier on the golf course. One way to develop trust is to ask for guidance by stating "what do I need to learn today" and then just open the book and see where the Goddess brings you!

 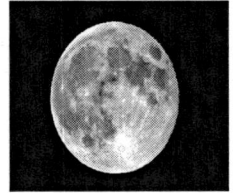

Part 1

Direction East-Element Air

Goddesses of Air –
Oya an African & Isis an Egyptian Goddess

- *Season: Spring*
- *Ceremony- Spring Equinox*
- *Quadrant of Day –Dawn*
- *Stage of Life-Birth*
- *Color and Race- Yellow*
- *Represents the Mind*

The direction of East is associated with New Beginnings, powers of the mind, intelligence, discernment, higher intuition and transformation. It is often the power of self-mastery through appropriate use of strength of will.

EAST - Air – Flight

Beginnings start in the east - from where the sun rises we begin a new dawn. Each day is a good new day with a fresh beginning, a new start. East is the direction of the physical body and newness including children and newborns. It is the time of change for all it is a new beginning. New ideas and seeing the light, Change. Spring is the season when all things begin to grow and awaken. Yellow is the path of Life, to begin the walk as a warrioress, a Golfing Goddess and to shine in all that you do. The sun rising in the east empowers each of us. The energy to do and to begin, the action of the mind and heart is here.

Yoga Poses for Air – pages **195-196**
Eagle, Pigeon, Butterfly, Half Locust

Chapter 1

Oya – African Air Goddess Transformation and Confidence

Oya's Attributes - A Goddess of storms, strong winds, fire and lightning; Ruler of the Marketplace.
Oya is a patron of women, especially of female intelligence and charm; she protects women traders in the marketplace.
The book of gods and goddesses. Eric Chaline.

Traditional African Praise of Oya -
*She burns like fire in the hearth, everywhere at once,
Tornado, quivering solid canopied trees
Great Oya, Yes.
Whirlwind masquerader, awakening
Courageously takes up her saber.*
-Judith Gleason

Goddess Oya representing the Front Nine

Hole 1 - Transformation

Zen Illustration-

I would like to begin the Chapter on transformation with a very ancient Zen story, about a lioness giving birth to a cub while she was jumping from one hillock to another hillock. The cub fell into a crowd of sheep and grew up amongst the sheep. There was no way for him to know that he was not a sheep -- he lived like the sheep, just eating grass and followed meekly just like all the other sheep.

Even eating grass he started becoming bigger than the sheep, longer, a beautiful specimen. But the sheep were not afraid; they never thought that he was dangerous. He had grown amongst them, they had relations with him, friends. Somebody mothered him, somebody was taking care of him; there was no question of being afraid. They were just concerned... what a strange kind of sheep! -- looks like a lion, but must be a natural mistake. And they were very happy to have him amongst them. While they moved in thousands in a crowd, he stood aloof in the middle of them.

One day an old lion saw this phenomenon and could not believe it. He had never seen any lion walking in a crowd of sheep. The moment sheep see a lion they start escaping -- it was a miracle.

The old lion went down to catch hold of the young lion. The sheep started running and the young lion also started running -- naturally. He believed he was a sheep.

But the old lion got hold of him. He started trembling, and the old lion said, "You idiot! You are trembling and weeping and crying and asking that you should be released because you want to join your group. There is something you don't know, it seems you are unaware, and I will not leave you unless I make you aware. You come with me!"

He dragged him to a nearby lake. The lake was silent -- no ripples, no wind was there. He took the young lion to the edge of the water and told him, "Look in the water. Look at my face and your face."

Instantaneously, from the young lion a roar came out. It was not any effort, it was simply the fact of seeing that he is a lion -- immediately a roar that resounded in faraway mountains. The old lion said, "My work is done. Now do you know who you are?"

The young lion thanked the old lion and said, "You have been very kind to me. Otherwise my whole life I would have lived chewing grass with the sheep, continuously afraid of being alone. You have given me a new birth."

We are never alone although that is not the meaning in this story the message is the recognition of your true being. I'm not sure when humans began to separate from nature and our true natural rhythms could it as people moved towards city life? It would seem that most of us have been conditioned to believe we are sheep and that all of us learn from a straight line of progress. On the contrary, this way of life creates an internal battle and is resulting in our greatest suffering. We will need to bring forth our roar, our hero, to help us move away from this conditioning and to connect back to the natural world and the lessons learned from the Circle of Life. It may seem like work at first because the roots of separation go down very deep but with awareness comes freedom. My message is connect and learn from the power of mother earth, not live in fear and try to conquer her.

To begin, Ladies let us replace Oya's saber from her African Praise with a golf club for our purposes. It is here that I will give you the secret of consistent golf that will give you the inner courage to play any course, with any of the so called "old boys club", gentry, clients or anywhere you may feel like you just don't belong. I am here to tell you, *Yes*, we are courageous, *Yes*, we do belong, Yes, we are golfing goddesses, *Yes*, we are good, *Yes*, we can be joyous while playing. *Yes*, we can learn from the earth we play upon. We can call upon Oya, to help us and maybe even begin to recognize her in ourselves. I will challenge your beliefs and bring you new insights just as the Goddess reveals them to me.

The golf course is still a playing field where many women feel intimidated. We have only been allowed recently to be part of this game with equal rights. Meaning that, on most courses we can have tee-off times whenever we like. But I still remember when I worked at a golf course in 1994 and we women were not allowed to book tee-off times Saturday mornings.

I believe there is enough room on the golf course for both genders; the thing that needs to change is everyone's perspective about woman golfers. I do see signs of change happening however and in the next couple of decades many won't remember it was an issue at all. I believe the similarity to women driving a golf ball is comparable to when women wanted to drive a car back in the 1960's. Girls today don't even know that there was so much resistance and jokes from men now, it is just a natural thing to do when you come of age for boys or girls.

Thankfully there have always been the smart innovative men who cater to women's needs and buying power that help with shifting perspectives. We can see evidence of this finally happening in ladies golf fashion, I don't know about you ladies but until recently I have thought women's golf wear was awful. To me it seemed men had dominance in the way we dressed because they didn't want distractions, sure women could dress sexy anywhere but on the golf course. As Goddesses we don't need play those games to win at golf. We just want to wear shorts and a tank top because they are comfortable for us and now the smart clothing companies are producing what we need.

Over the years many women have started the game just to give it up again and I want to encourage those to try the game one more time as a Golf Goddess. If while playing any of you do encounter some dinosaur thinking, than I will arm you with some knowledge that I found on the Internet. History shows women have been playing golf for a long time and it's up to us women to remind men of this fact, that their dearly beloved game had the help of a woman to bring it to popularity.

The game of golf was developed in Scotland in the early 16th Century and had its advocates in the Royal family of Scotland. It had been introduced to France along with the entourage that went with Mary Queen of Scots to the French court. This event marked the beginning of the spread of golf to its current global status as a sport.

Mary, Queen of Scots was a notable player. So keen was her interest in the game that she fell foul of the Church for playing golf only a few days after the murder of her second husband, Lord Darnley, rather than demonstrating a proper amount of time in mourning following his murder and death. While in France Mary played golf as one of her favorite activities, helping spread the early popularity of the game.

http://www.artsales.com/topics/golf_history/historyofGolf.htm

If you ever find yourself in a scenario that I am about to relate, you can use the above information, which I did, although I added bit more flair. Like the year, it just came out of my mouth; so don't quote me on it. I was taking an older gentleman client golfing at a semi-private course and we were paired up with two young men who were members. We were at the tee-box waiting for the group ahead to finish and one of the Guy's said, "I heard that GOLF means Gentleman Only Ladies Forbidden." I replied, "Did you know that in the year 1635, Mary, Queen of Scots played a golf game after her husband was murdered"? That shut him up. So why would he say this in the first place? Well I found out they were just like little boys trying to throw me off balance, teasing, ribbing me; I felt like I was back home with my three brothers. Then this client who I thought was a gentleman gets into the same kind of mood.

He starts wanting to bet, only with me though, and stupid bets like, "I bet you five bucks I can out drive you." Well, we are on the 15th hole by now and he has out driven me each shot. So, what I am going to do - lose my money to him on purpose? I don't think so. I stayed empowered and said, "No thank you" in a soft and kind voice and played my shots from a calm centered place, knowing I would not do business with this man nor play golf with him again.

That day I thought about women giving up and if it's because they often experience men acting like boys, I can understand it. But ladies I'm here to tell you Never Give Up! Especially for using the game of golf as a business tool, if you aren't using it already, then begin as soon as you can. There are many scenarios of women who have a good product or services and haven't been able to make the sales like their male competitors and the one ingredient they were lacking was taking their clients golfing. You can get to know a person more intimately by spending four hours golfing than an hour over lunch. People buy from people they trust and golf can be viewed as a faster tool to build relationships with others. Because of this it has also become a great networking tool.

I've heard of some companies who use the game of golf before hiring an executive. They want to see how a potential employee plays the game of golf, how they react under pressure, if they are honest, and have integrity. Using the game of golf as a mirror to the game of life by gaining knowledge about someone's personality is seen as a powerful business tool.

When people ask what I do, and I say that I teach yoga for golf, I can get more clients. It is funny how people have reacted over the years when I do my stretches on the first tee. They see me as a committed golfer who is in charge of my game. And it makes a good impression and it used to intimidate golfers as well giving me an advantage. So if you want to boost your sales and your game, begin playing and practicing these concepts to the best of your ability.

If you have never played before then your transformation from a non-golfer to a golfer can begin before even hitting a ball.

We can call upon Oya, "The Queen of the Wind of Changes" to help us transform from a good player to a great player consistently, a great player into a champion!

"We don't so much conquer the golf course but ourselves."

The golf course is one place where changes do occur every day just look at the pin placement for example. This evidence can be a good thing to get used to in our lives by remembering, the only thing constant is change. By tapping into a very powerful tool, your mind, you can co-create the changes you want. Let us begin to develop an exercise program not only for your body but for your mind as well we begin this with the principles of Raja yoga. Your mind can work for you or against you. We are going to develop an exercise program for the mind to help re-train and re- program the sub-conscious mind to utilize it as much as possible.

Here in the West we are taught to be very left brained, logical, rational, linear thinkers. In the East they are more in touch with their right brain, the intuition, creativity, emotions. We will learn to create a balance between our intuition and our intellect.

So where do we start? There is a word in Yoga called Karma which means cause and effect. Thoughts are the cause and the effect is what shows up in our lives or in other words our experiences. We can look at our minds like a computer, our thoughts are the data going into the computer and then we view that data on the screen. Negative thoughts can be viewed as a virus so the screen is not clear or it shuts down altogether. This same analogy can be applied to our golf game the thoughts we say to ourselves produce the experience we see on the screen of the golf course. To grasp this concept on a deep level you will need to find a willing participant to do this easy but very powerful experiment with. The person doesn't have to be a golfer and you can do it without a club in your hand. I am just outlining the steps the way I teach it to a class.

Kinesiology Test
1. Hold out your strongest arm straight in front of you at shoulder height, and your other hand could be holding a golf club or down at your side.
2. You will say out loud 5 times "I hate this club", shake out your arm and say another 5 times "I play weak with this club".
3. Your partner simultaneously places their hand on top of your out stretched arm and tries to push your arm down with one hand, while you are saying your statements and the partner is using their other hand they will count to 5 for you each time.
4. You will resist this pressure as if you had your hand against a wall
5. After this is said both statements for a total of 10 times, shake out your arm, and hold it up again, use the same procedure as before but now state out loud that "I LOVE my golf club" 5 times and then state an other 5 times "I play strong with this club"
6. Just for good measure one last time say out loud 5 times " I play weak with this club".

Then you can change partners. Pretty powerful stuff, don't you agree?
You have just been introduced to your sub-conscious mind, and you can see for yourself the truth that it doesn't judge, it just reacts to what you tell it to do.

Whatever you do, think or say comes back to you just like a boomerang; there is no good or bad, no judgment, it just is.

Now this is very important lesson and it is one I would like you to keep foremost in your consciousness, if we use the analogy of a computer once more, this information works best by storing it on the desktop so it is easily accessible. Do not think of this as insignificant and store it away. By working on our inner game we see the effects on the screen of the golf course much quicker, then only working on the outer game.

When my students come to class, I do the arm experiment by first asking them to bring in their worst club the week before. When they arrive I ask if they brought in their worst club; they agree and tell me why. I then say to them, "It is no different than any other club in your bag. It is only your belief that it doesn't work well for you." Just because you had an off game with that club those thoughts stayed with you and then you manifest that over and over. Change the belief and you change how the club will perform for you. I find it interesting that out of hundreds of students that I have taught this to, there have been only a few who said they like all their clubs equally. I am still surprised at this and if you are one of those players, congratulations, because it is a rare quality.

The golf club is just a thing, but it becomes an extension of you and your thoughts on the golf course. Hmmmm . . . I wonder if I need to add another example? Sure why not. When I came to the conclusion that the club is an extension, I remembered fishing in my younger years. I reflected on the fact that when I really wanted to catch a fish I never would, but when I was relaxed and focused on the scenery and not on fishing, I inevitably caught more.

I realized that the fishing rod was an extension of my feelings and the fish were sensitive enough to feel the vibrations of the rod. When I wanted a fish, I was holding the rod tight, because internally I had tension of trying too hard. The fish wouldn't take the bait with the tension involved. When I was relaxed and not paying attention the rod was not an obstacle to the fish and the bait. Who knows what the line and bait look like down below to the fish. But it was the same every time. Relaxed me, relaxed line, and more fish. In golf I discovered the same holds true the club acts like an extension of my thoughts and feelings, relaxed me, relaxed club, more power, we will explore the subject that relaxation equals power further on.

You will discover if you don't like the way you are playing your game on any given day then you probably need to change your thinking. Think on this quote:

> "We know that habits are in control, the question is
> are they friend or are they foe."

Are you aware of good habits while playing, and can you recognize undesirable habits while playing?

I often give my students a challenge.

I ask them to play a game of golf by themselves and begin to notice what thoughts they are saying to themselves. Imagine after a few holes of becoming aware of those thoughts that this is a person you are paired up with. Notice if this is an encouraging partner or not. The feedback is usually one of surprise but not in a pleasant way. Usually people realize that after making a bad shot that they'll say "I'm such an idiot" and they think they will say this a couple of times throughout the game. They are not prepared for all the other negative thoughts or how fast the game goes downhill once they become aware. I tell them, "Don't despair, that was only a temporary necessity". Because once golfers become aware of their thoughts they are on the first step to changing them. Most people I know like to see themselves as good, kind and generous and are surprised that they do not offer these same qualities to themselves. It seems to be easier to give encouragement and be kind to others while being our own worst enemy.

When golfers are giving me their feedback on their solitude golfing day, I ask them, "If your thoughts were a real person how many times would you golf with this person?" They wouldn't, and they want to know how to change.

Are you brave enough to take the same challenge? If you can't play alone, then you could ask a trusted friend to help you out by being your mirror. They repeat back to you every time you say a degrading word about yourself. You can also make marks on the scorecard of all the ones you say out loud and all the ones you say in your mind. Know that there is always room for improvement. What I mean by that is if you say one encouraging word for every three non-encouraging words you can begin to change the ratio.

Again this exercise shows that whatever you tell yourself your body carries out perfectly. This is very helpful knowledge if we belong to a country club or even if we play the same golf course many times throughout the season. If we bring the past into the moment by saying to ourselves, "Oh, here we are at the third hole. I always bogey the third hole." Guess what? You'll do it again, it becomes a self-fulfilling prophecy. We need to look at each game as a fresh new experience and not bring the past into the present so we can be open to creating anew each and every time we play. One of the best ways to stay in the moment is to have what in Zen is called a beginner's mind each and every time we play golf. Especially if you are a member of a golf course it is easy to keep recreating the same game or the same holes over and over. If it's a birdie at a specific hole, that's great, keep it up, but if it's a bogey, then it's time to create a new outcome with a beginner's mind which is open and full of acceptance.

I heard somewhere that the three main stresses in golf are all because of expectations:

1. Expectations of yourself.
2. Other people's expectations of you.
3. Your expectations of other people.

One of my favorite quotes that I help my students to use in helping overcome expectations is from the book *"The Knight in the Rusty Armor"* by *Robert Fisher* is:

"When we learn to accept instead of expect we will have fewer disappointments".

Many golfers approach a golf course already stressed out. Emotions are flying high, tremendous risks are taken without a second thought, tantrums are thrown and irrational strategy seems to guide their actions. Many complain throughout the whole game and at the end of the day when they come into the clubhouse and you ask how their game was they reply, "I had a terrible game". They began on a downward spiral and continued going down.

Arriving at a golf course with the mind set of saying to yourself, "okay today I am not going to judge I am going to just accept whatever happens." This takes practice but it is so freeing. We can have preferences about certain things but not be rigid and try to control. Control can be a sure recipe for disappointment, maybe not right away but over time it creates huge internal tension. So you see, you can actually create the game in your mind with your thoughts, images and feelings even before you swing a club.

Do you know if you are consciously creating great golf? Once again I say awareness is the key. You just experienced one exercise in awareness. Let us go into it even deeper. I want to illustrate a short but powerful story I read from an email, which I have slightly altered for golfers.

Story: One day a grandmother took her granddaughter golfing. While they were waiting at one of the holes, the grandmother said to her granddaughter, "Lynn, when I am playing golf it is as if I have two cats fighting inside me; one is yowling anger, doubt, frustration, fear and the other is purring with contentment, joy, confidence, gratitude." Lynn thinks about this for a minute and then turns to her Grandmother and asks, "Which one wins?" and her grandmother replies, "The one I feed."

When I tell the above story to my class I get some laughs immediately and some people pause and think, then respond with nods of their heads or with a chuckle. Without awareness most of us are so used to an inner critic that we don't even know that something has to be turned off or the channel to be changed to a more positive and productive one. Can you tell by the way your life is lived right now what kind of thoughts you are repeatedly feeding yourself? You can pretty much be guaranteed they will be of the same sort of nature while playing golf. The great thing is if you become your own best friend on the golf course it will naturally happen in your daily life as well. In a much easier transition than vice versa, become your best friend in golf and it will spill into every other area of your life. You see, to overcome the habits in daily life will take longer as they are older and stronger than the ones you have acquired while playing golf. What has been helpful to me is a line I saw by author Kent Nerburn, *"The world is made, not out of problems, but of dreams."* Which one wins? So Goddesses I encourage you to feed your dreams many times throughout the day and the habit of feeding your problems will slip away naturally. Not release our habits by stilling the mind completely. Then what are we to do? This guru recommends that thought-waves of anger, fear and delusion, must be first overcome by replacing them with higher, non-painful thought–waves. We must oppose these, with thoughts with love, generosity and truth."

Let us go back for a moment to Patanjali the Father of Yoga and his teachings "He says that we do not release our habits by stilling the mind completely. Then what are we to do? This guru recommends that thought-waves of anger, fear and delusion, must be first overcome by replacing them with higher, non-painful thought–waves. We must oppose these, with thoughts with love, generosity and truth."

This takes practice, especially while playing golf. So before we can still the mind, we must replace our thoughts and our habits, with more positive ones. Sounds simple right?

The simplest solution I have found is in the Law of Attraction. Everything what we put out comes back. Through the native tradition I was taught same principle said slightly different, "be careful what you put into your circle." So to make and create better shots and results, we must raise our vibrations while playing golf. It is not a sport that we can use sound to help us, unless we have made a hole-in-one. Sound is a great way to move energy just look at fans in a stadium and how much better players do when they are cheered, or how hard it is to overcome the boo's and still win. The teams that keep winning no matter what crowd they are in front of have transformed themselves and have strong spirits.

At the moment we can't use sound to transform us to happier more upbeat players. Although we can use gratitude, appreciation is what attracted me to the Native Path my deep love of nature is reflected in their ancient ways of love, respect and gratitude for nature. Gratefulness brings us more to our hearts and then the good feelings help our playing. My suggestion is, as soon as you can, go play a Gratitude Game. Imagine approaching your playing partners and saying "I would like your help on an assignment I have to do. The next game we play, we are to focus on what we are grateful for that day." Now you don't ask them to observe any effects, but I want you to be the observer for them and for you. Notice if the energy changes like happier feelings, and conversation, more relaxed body language, balls start finding the holes in amazing ways for you to be more grateful for. Then notice the conversation at the end of the game, this would be the time to point out the differences if they haven't noticed already. This theme Gratitude can be used many times and in many ways, I leave the creation up to you. Whatever you are grateful for will show up more in your life. A few times you will read that I ask you to feel good feelings one of the best ways to bring you to the 'feeling' is through gratitude lists.

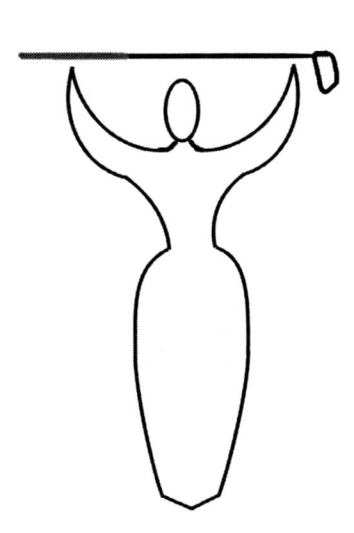

Goddess Oya representing the Back Nine

Hole 10 - Confidence

Confidence begins with Affirmations for your Golf-Esteem

Definition of Affirmations: to make Firm what is already true or has the potential to become true.

One way to use this page is to close your eyes and ask your wise inner self what message you need to work on. Move your hand over the pages and then point your finger down, open your eyes and repeat that phrase over and over for the next few days. You may have heard it takes 21 days to replace an old habit. It takes saying a new belief one hundred thousand times before it becomes a life-long habit. You won't possibly overstate your phrase.

Two ways to increase your new belief is by saying your affirmations, using the element of air to speak the words aloud, the other is by repeating the affirmations in front of a mirror. A final ingredient for the fastest results in cutting that 100,000 in half is to include your positive emotions such as happiness, playfulness, and gratitude.

"A bad attitude is worse than a bad swing"
– Payne Stewart

Come, Be Golfing Goddesses!

I am a peak performer
I believe in my game and ability to score
I am a great putter
I am self-disciplined
I drive the ball well
I recover quickly from temporary setbacks
I am confident in my short game
I trust myself to do my best
I am in great shape and stronger then ever
I have focused awareness for every shot

I am patient
My golf game is fun
I always learn from my mistakes
I always trust my first instinct when selecting a club
I am taking more risks everyday
Whether you think you can or you think you can't, your right (Henry Ford)
I posses everything I need to create a great golf game
I am confident
I am relaxed and calm
I am a great golfer
I am a calm and composed golfer
I use every challenge as an opportunity to grow
It's not what happens, but how I respond that creates a great game
I produce quality results with excellence and ease
I am aware that my thoughts are creating my game -good or bad
I say only positive words to myself
I am incredible Goddess energy
I relax and let go
Bring on the Joy, bring on the Love
My best shots are chip shots
I am always delighted with the results I produce
I am disciplined
My tee shots are always accurate
I forgive myself and move on
I love to stretch my body
I am supported by the Goddess in every way
I am committed to achieving my goals
I visualize all of my goals as complete and achieved now

Please don't skip over this simple exercise. I tested it out with my partner who at the time hadn't become a golfer yet. He didn't want to participate but finally with enough encouragement on my part he did. His finger landed on, "I am relaxed and calm", his wise mind led him to what he needed at the time, which he thought was very cool because the reason he didn't want to do it in the first place is because most of the affirmations are statements for a golfer.

> *"We are what we repeatedly do.*
> *Excellence then, is not an act, but a habit.*
> *"- Aristotle*

In Napoleon Hill's the timeless book *Think & Grow Rich*, he studied wealthy men for 20 years and in his findings he came across this secret and beneficial fact, *"Repetition of affirmation of order to your sub-conscious mind is the only known method of voluntary development of the emotion of faith."*

The same results are known as a mantra found Bhakti yoga, which uses chanting or singing a phrase over and over, this has been used for thousands of years, and the Goddess tradition says, "that which is repeated, gains density and becomes tangible."

I experimented with the truth of gaining faith through affirmations years ago with the help of a book called *The Magic of Believing* by Claude Bristol, a book that literally fell off the bookshelf in the library. There were many useful examples of the power of auto- suggestion to bridge the gap of believing that you can create your life the way you desire it. (of course the Universe may step in and put some obstacles and detours up but remember if the Goddess brings you to it, she will bring you through it). The following experiment from this book is what I believe helped me gain faith that we are powerful beings and it can be the same for anyone. You will be able to start manifesting a parking spot right out front of where you are going. Before you leave the house say out loud, "I will park right in front of the bank." (or wherever). Now Claude assures us, and as someone who knows it works, I assure you as well. Don't give up if it doesn't happen immediately. Just keep practicing until one day it happens, than you will get excited and want to keep practicing. The excitement brings more of the experiences to you until one day you are confident that you will always get a parking spot out front of where you are going. Because as soon as you get in the car you state what you want, you believe it will happen, and the Universe says "Yes" to your command and delivers back to you what you believe. This simple exercise brings belief to the forefront and then confidence begins to builds as a result. If you would rather relate it to golf, begin to say "I always find golf balls." You will begin to see more golf balls show up even if you are not on the golf course!

Faith is such a great unshakeable confidence it is worth the effort of repeating affirmations

A story in confidence comes from teaching a junior golfer who came for some private yoga for golf classes one spring and he continued with them all summer long. He had just completed his first year at college on a golf scholarship. He had lost confidence in his ability to play. He was a good player but a bad thinker. After going through the list of the above affirmations and seeing which ones he believed and didn't believe, I asked him which one he thought would help him the most. He didn't believe, "I recover quickly from temporary setbacks." He said that was his biggest problem at the moment. He couldn't recover and so he was losing faith in himself. I then asked him what he believed to be his biggest strength while playing and it was a different affirmation than I had here. He told me "I put the best when under pressure."

Well, I thought, we are half way there if that is his belief. Because of the power of that statement he will be back on top of his game in no time. You see he had a great deal of confidence before he went to college, but after seeing all the good players he became intimidated and began to lose faith in himself. So, by getting inside his head and finding out what he was thinking and believing, we worked on correcting the problem, which left his body clear to do what it already knew how to do, which was play great golf.

Now let me tell you how he began to improve by using these two affirmations. If we think about them as autosuggestions we see it is a form of self-hypnosis. The first autosuggestion was just a flimsy thought, which is how all habits begin. He didn't really believe it but because we did the kinesiology test in this book which proved how his strong words equaled a strong performance in his body so he was willing to repeat this affirmation over and over. In a short time he began to experience that he was bouncing back easily from setbacks until one day he noticed a consistency in how quickly he could recover, and by the end of the summer he had faith in himself to recover and was not in fear or anxious in tournaments like he had been before.

With his tension removed he began winning more. Now the interesting part of his second suggestion was that it surpassed just being a belief and became a deeper knowing within him. He knew he putted the best under pressure because he had seen the results before we even talked about it. But by the end of the summer with his continuous repetition it became a strong, steel cable to pull him to victory. He was a confident putter.

I encourage you to read this next statement over and over if you need any more evidence on the importance of the simple task of repeating affirmations. Napoleon Hill assures us, "Repetition of affirmation of orders to your subconscious mind is the only known method of voluntary development of the emotion of faith."

This faith, this belief in yourself and your desires, has been practiced in India for thousands of years with Bhakti Yoga which uses mantra's a repetition of words or phrases to bring about the desires of devotees. This power in our day and age can be viewed in the form of advertising.

If we want further proof of the power of suggestion we only have look at advertising to help us with this concept. Think about how many times they repeat a message when it is some new idea they want to get across. They play it as a continuous tape over and over and over until the flimsy idea becomes a belief. For example, some years ago the message was to have whiter teeth; this concept was everywhere we turned - TV, stores, computer, radio, billboards - and what was the underlying message? You are not a worthy person if your teeth aren't white. Think about how you were swayed by this? Yes, there are still some commercials out there, but not as many as there were when the concept was new. Did they create a habit in people? Is the concept so embedded in the conscious mind that the choice is so simple that when buying toothpaste you naturally purchase the one with whitening in it?

The example of the bombardment advertising companies use to sell you a new idea, which is a new product, goes back to what I mentioned earlier - you cannot overstate your affirmations. Just as my client did, I suggest you use a statement you already believe in and one that you need to work on, to test the results yourself. See which one begins working quicker for you. Usually it will be the one you already believe in and that is because you have already created good feelings around it from gaining results. Think about what good feelings you would have if you knew that you putted the best under pressure. I can't stress this enough, the more good emotions you add to your affirmations the quicker the results. You need to trust your body to know how to make the shot. You have made great shots! So if you get your mind out of the way your body can do what it knows how to do effortlessly and consistently. One of the best analogies I've heard for this is driving a standard car. When you are first learning to drive you are focused on the mechanics of learning. You are steering the car, pushing in the clutch and changing gears at the same time. You keep repeating the instructions over and over in your mind. With repeated repetition you build muscle memory and then move from your conscious mind to your sub-conscious mind, which acts out those instructions effortlessly.

The body is functioning on automatic pilot and you can begin to add the view and scenery to your drive because your mind is free of instructions. This is the stage we want to attain in golf to have the mind free of the instructions and to be able to focus on the scenery, the course lay out and what is happening in the moment. The concepts of belief, positive affirmations, and becoming your own coach have been in my teachings from day one. These concepts were hard for most people to grasp ten years ago because the main belief about golf was learning the mechanics. This was quite out of the box for them. This path I have been on educating golfers about yoga for golf has tested me many, many times to be my own encouraging coach. It has been a long journey, with many obstacles along the way, mostly because I have not made the money I thought I would and sometimes it was just living with the barest of things and all the sacrifices for what I now see is my personal calling. I have lived with proof that trusting totally in the Divine may not always bring me what I want right away but I am always provided instantly with what I need. I left the world of working for money when I left the bartending. It fed my pocketbook but not my soul. I used to joke in the early days of teaching, I said, "I knew I was destined to serve spirit, I was just confused for a while and served the wrong spirits to people."

It wasn't the spirit of drinks that my being wanted me to focus on it was helping others to develop their own spirits. There have been a few jobs here and there but I have never truly gone back to the workforce since the conception of my business. So saying this, every theme in this book I have walked many times again and again on and off the course.

When the new science, quantum physics began educating the public, I grasped it immediately, I realized this is what I had been teaching all along. That is because this is the first time in history that science and spirituality are now speaking the same language. One great movie on quantum physics is called *What the Bleep do we Know*, which I recommend for my more advanced students. I have learned it is useful to surround oneself with books, tapes, movies on the same subject matter when first incorporating it for support and to help us stay confident it is easy to go back to the same old habits otherwise. The more you open yourself to new concepts by different sources the more you can recognize when these principles are happening in your life. While I was writing this book throughout 2006 -2008 a movie came out called *The Secret*, about the Laws of Attraction.

Although I personally didn't like this movie as much as the first one I mentioned, I am grateful for it because it has made my classes more enjoyable to teach since the people who have seen it can grasp my concepts more easily then my past students. I actually used to get headaches from teaching some classes in the early years because the students were trying so hard to understand.

To reiterate again, the more exposed to reading, listening, and watching material on the same subject, the more "good food" you develop for your mind and soul. There are Man Made Laws and Natures Laws. With more knowledge of both, the better you

can decide the best course for your life. I have discovered that this is a life-long journey of learning and we are always still becoming.

As we learn more about the Goddesses we see ourselves in them - the shadow and the light. We live in a world of paradoxes, of opposites. We have been taught to ignore or push away the shadow side of ourselves. In the Viking Runes, the first rule is to 'Know Thyself'. In Jungian philosophy, it is the repressed parts that are not safe to show the world – to be a Goddess of the storm, a tornado, how unlady like. This puritan belief is imbedded in our sub-conscious minds.

As we transform our beliefs through the use of golf and goddesses we set ourselves free. "The truth will set you free". Take responsibility for the way you create your game. No one can do it for you. They can only point the way. Only you control what goes on in your head, positive or negative. As Shakespeare once said, "There is nothing good or bad, but thinking makes it so."

I had a second vision from Mother Mary in 2000 and in this vision she informed me that I was to begin teaching people to control their thoughts, this was because time was speeding up and what people thought about is going to happen at a faster rate, good or bad.

I was inspired to produce a golf CD that had the golf affirmations on it to help golfers along. This concept is simple but not easy. It takes work to keep repeating affirmations and I found many students would not continue when they left a session because they weren't exposed to them anymore. So by having the c.d. it did the work for them.

One thing I have learned about positive thinking and being clear on your desire and affirming what you want - it is a life- long practice. For me it's like taking vitamins. When I start to feel good I stop, and then I feel tired again and have to start my vitamins once more. When I feel confident and in the flow by saying my affirmations I will stop and then I have to begin again when I'm not in sync. Fear and doubt can never be completely overcome; they can shrink to little seeds and seem to grow when affirmations are stopped, especially when you are trying something new. This is definitely a discipline. After reading the quote below, see if you recognize the truth in it.

"WATCH YOUR THOUGHTS
THEY BECOME WORDS,

WATCH YOUR WORDS
THEY BECOME HABIT,

WATCH YOUR HABIT
FOR IT BECOMES YOUR CHARACTER,

WATCH YOUR CHARACTER
FOR IT BECOMES YOUR ....DESTINY."
- Buddha

When moving and going through my paper work, I found all kinds of affirming messages I have written out for myself over the years. This evidence reminded me that

I do use the tools and have all along, but when I take them for granted it's harder to recognize this fact, so it was a nice awareness to find the affirmations. One that I would like to share that I used to have written on a white board in my kitchen for a long time is; "Good morning, _____ This is the Goddess Speaking, I will be taking care of all your worries today, and I won't be needing your help."

I am once again consistent with my affirmations and I find it easier to be in a state of gratefulness because of events spontaneously occurring faster and faster. I believe that once started on the path of affirmations there is a pathway developed in your mind, so if you stop and then start again you are not starting back at square one.

You just continue where you left off with built up faith and quick responses. When the results are quick, gratitude becomes a natural reaction. Gratitude helps me and can help you stay and feel confident all day long. To reiterate once again - when you start saying the affirmations of creating your life, you then watch for the signs along the way.

When they begin to appear, be ever so grateful. By noticing them you are telling your subconscious mind that they are what you really want. The more you put your attention on something, the more it expands because you literally become a magnet for what you want. You can ask for whatever you want, good or bad. It doesn't matter, the subconscious doesn't judge, it just begins going to work on what you ask for.

It is very important to begin training yourself to start paying attention and gaining control of the negative because there is a witness always listening even if you are not. I noticed that I was giving myself a mixed message for so many years. I keep reading about follow your passion and the money would come. I was a single mother and an owner of a yoga studio but even though I was doing what I loved I was in fear. The mixed messages brought mixed money. It would depend on what feelings where stronger. I would say I wanted more money and then I would only bemoan what I didn't have and that I wasn't going to get to pay this bill or that bill. Then when the bill was about to arrive I would have a temper tantrum with the Goddesses and say things in a demanding way. "Where is the money? I know you can help me. I need the money. You have done it in the past. I need it done again."

The last command had a belief so strong attached to it the money would arrive from some unexpected source. I found when you go beyond belief to a deep knowing, you have what you want almost instantly which is so cool, and then you know you are co- creating and always taken care of. Instead of being scared about the unknown it is going back to being child-like and living in the wonder. I now have begun to say to myself, "I wonder how the Goddess will provide for us. I wonder how the Goddess will manifest my dreams. And the new one which happens once a week is. "I wonder what we will get for free." Something always shows up because we have no attachment, idea, or even really have any time invested for when it does. Then we say Thank you and immediately ask, "I wonder what the Universe will bring us next for free." My old habit was to state my intention to have something, and then say I don't see how I will get it. Why do we live in fear? Is it conditioning, advertising, is it because everyone else is doing it? There must be some truth in the saying "misery loves company".

In our society, in the west anyway, I notice that we can have a great day and then one thing bad happens and that is what we focus on and tell others about. It is the same with golf. We tell the war tales, not the great shots we had. Some people feel that if they say the positive things they are bragging and it will turn others off. One thing we could practice is what my mother used to say, and maybe yours did too; "If you don't have anything nice to say, don't say anything at all." Boy, we could have a lot of quiet public places if no one went around complaining. So being aware and keeping vigilant attention on keeping the inner critic at bay is an on-going process. Don't let the old voices get you down. They only have power if you listen to them. Of course, I find I teach what I most need to learn. Experts tell us that exercising helps keep our mood high as it helps in the release of endorphins the feel good hormones. To add the practice of yoga or walking the golf course to affirmations can have you feelin' fine most of the time.

- If your inner critic does get you down, ask yourself some questions:
- Is this thought really the truth? How does this thought serve me?
- What is more a productive counter thought I can say instead?

Chapter 2

Isis – Egyptian Air Goddess Pranayama and Relaxation

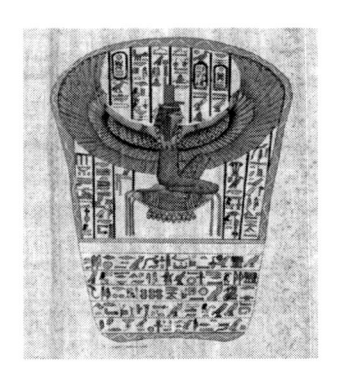

Myth - Isis was a popular mother goddess, her lap being held to represent the throne of Egypt. She was adept at healing and magic and Egyptians believed that she could change her physical form at will. Isis was sister-consort of Osiris and helped gather his body parts after Seth had scattered them across Egypt. She also ensured his resurrection by gently flapping her wings to raise a breeze that enabled Osiris to Breathe.

– Book by Eric Chaline

Attributes - As a divine healer, Isis shared the secrets of healing and preparation of medical potions with her priestesses. Isis is also credited for bringing us the secrets of law and agriculture. If you ask anyone that esteems Isis to the role of goddess in this present age; you will surely hear them proclaim that Isis holds life in her hands. Isis, with her ability to breathe life into something once dead, is worshipped today as she has been for centuries.

Come, Be Golfing Goddesses!

Goddess Isis representing the Front Nine

Hole 2 - Pranayama

One attribute given to the Goddess Isis is the Breath of Life. Let us call upon Isis to breathe life and vitality into us. New life into a dead golf game, to let go of an old game, breathe new life into it. Maybe it's a dead career - than play golf to be out in nature, breathe in the fresh air and bring creative thinking back to work.

In this chapter I am going to continue the theme of transformation by using the best tool I know of to date, called pranayama. Prana means life force and yama means control. What you will be learning is how to gain breath control for the most life force for your body. I feel these breathing techniques are the most important practices in this whole book! They may take a while to develop but they are a life-long skill and well worth the practice. Air is vital to our lives. Think about how long you can go without air compared to any other source that gives us life. We can go weeks without eating, days without water but only minutes without air.

Yogis hold the belief that air is our most essential food and that one should seek to breathe air of the highest nutritional value. The most vitalizing air that is charged with prana or life force is by the sea, large open spaces, lakes and mountains.

The longer and slower one breathes the longer their life span increases. Slow deep breathing is conducive to meditative states of consciousness and happier lives. With the combined power of using your breath when you swing the club you will have consistent and outstanding shots. The more you develop your lungs the better your drives will be. Also you will become a less nervous player and a steadier putter.

We are about to learn how to make the unconscious, conscious. First we learn to breathe properly indoors, with the intent to remember it is best to do this outside.

Pranayama/ Breath Control Benefits –
- It increases the body's capacity to absorb and store prana.

- We obtain mastery and control over our prana body, our energy body, vital body that stores the psychic body and mental body. This implies that by practicing Pranayama we gain a deep insight into letting go of all psychic burdens, dissolving all Karma, and purifying the mind.

- It provides a direct avenue of communication to the Higher Self, going beyond the mind and deeper than words.

- It balances all systems of polarity in the body, i.e. Sympathetic and Parasympathetic nervous systems, right and left-brain hemispheres and their functions, body and mind with feelings and emotions, inner male and inner female within us.

- It induces relaxation, steadiness of mind, and bliss and creates calmness and clarity.

Are we really Breathing?

I had an 87 year old beginner client whose niece signed him up for some personal Yoga For Golf classes. When she asked him how his first class went, he told her "I learned how to breathe." This may sound incredible to some people. How can you teach anyone to breathe isn't the most natural thing in our lives you may ask?

Especially for someone who has been breathing their whole life. As mentioned briefly, in India they call conscious breathing, Pranayama – Breath Control.

A common practice for many new students is to be retrained to breathe properly, unless they had previous training such as a stress management course. Many wellness-based programs now use the basis of yogic breathing because of its calming effects. Now, not only do you use the breath to be calm, but to help with holding the poses longer. It is the holding of a pose that brings the elasticity to the body, so, in every beginner yoga session I must begin with teaching the students how to breathe the yogic breath, because breathing and the yoga postures go hand in hand. If you are not breathing while doing yoga you are tense and tight. A person needs to be relaxed to go deeper into the yoga poses. I inform my classes at the beginning that all breathing is done in and out of the nose unless it is a specific pranayama we are practicing. When asked "Why can't I exhale from my mouth?" (which is a retraining in itself.), I say, "for two reasons." First when you exhale from your mouth, it is not a complete exhale, meaning not all of the air is expelled.

This is particularly evident while certain yoga poses. This statement is beneficial in two ways, one being that when you exhale from the nose it is a longer and fuller breath, and then the body automatically takes in a deeper inhale, bringing more oxygen to the body.

Secondly in essence, the breath is your true teacher. It tells you when to come out of a pose. When we are holding a pose and start off with deep breaths, we are in a good range, not going too far into the stretch. If you are in a stretch and your breath is short and tight, it means you have gone into it too far and need to back out of it until your breath flows more smoothly and deeply. While holding the pose, the body will give you the signal (when that deep breath becomes shallower) that it is time to come out of the stretch. Your breath and body are giving the signal that you are working too hard and it's time to rest for a moment.

Now, paradoxically, when the body starts to become more flexible and is used to holding the poses you can use the deep exhale to go a deeper into a stretch. The same principles apply to golf. Over the years I have asked many people if they breathe when they swing a club. Most answer they don't know and some simply say no. If you are not breathing while swinging the club, your muscles stay tight and tense; hence shorter muscles, shorter swing. For longer more fluid drives one must breathe.

It is also a great way to keep the body relaxed. One time I was going for a meeting with a well-known golf pro and a man came up to her and said, "How do I relax when I am swinging the club? I know that I need to but I don't know how?" She replied, "Well if you know you need to, than just do it." And she walked away with me tagging behind because I didn't have the courage at the time to speak up. It has stuck with me ever since as a missed opportunity to help someone, so I want you to understand that it has been through experimenting, first by myself and then with my students - the correlation of breathing into yoga poses and breathing into your golf swings really works. Not only do we gain a more rhythmic swing but we gain more yards to our drives and more vitality and stamina for all 18 holes and also have less pain in our bodies at the end of the game, since deep breathing helps eliminate lactic acid build up.

The first breath we learn is the Diaphragmatic Breath, or simply called Belly Breathing. This breath seems backwards to most people as I am told because it is opposite to most fitness programs.

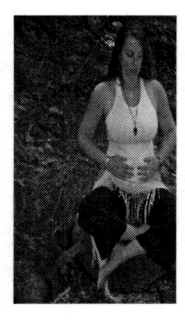

Belly Breathing

Breathing from your belly, or the diaphragmatic breath, does not involve the upper part of your body at all.

1. First place your hands lightly upon your belly; it is important to have a straight back if sitting up and to always breathe through the nose with both the inhale and exhale.
2. Inhale and imagine your abdomen is a balloon that you are filling with air and feel the belly expand.
3. When you exhale, purposely release all the air out completely, deflating the balloon and imagining your belly button going back towards your spine.

Begin the practice with five of these breaths.

To get this sensation even more deeply ingrained it is helpful to lie on a hard surface such as the floor in what is called crocodile pose. Place one hand on top of the other and place your head on your hands. Now breathing the belly breath you would inhale and push your abdomen on the floor, and when you exhale you pull your navel in towards your spine.

This is our natural way of breathing. If you were to watch an infant breathe you would notice the abdomen moving up and down with each breath in and out. Or if you ever played a winded instrument like the flute, you should have been taught to breathe from the diaphragm. This is the beginning place that will lead up to the full yogic complete breath. In other words, if I was to ask you to take a deep breath I would want it to begin from the belly. Most people are shallow breathers; this is a vicious circle to be in. When we breathe only from the upper chest it keeps the body tense and nervous, and when the body is tense and nervous one tends to breathe shallow. To break this chain we need to learn and utilize the belly breathing.

Breathing, like everything else, becomes habitual. Experts tell us it takes 21 days to break a habit, so here is an exercise for in the car. Whenever you are driving and you are at a red light, this will be your practice place. Push your belly out on the inhale, pull it inwards for the exhale. If you don't drive, think of an another activity where you can practice breathing from your belly like every time you are on the computer and you are waiting for something to open.

Over the years I have added this homework for my classes since many people find this breath hard to grasp, especially trying to learn new Yoga moves and breathing simultaneously. We are bringing our attention to an unconscious movement like breathing to train it to become a mindful act. So how did we move away from our natural way of breathing, and why don't many of my students want to practice the belly breath? They worry about gaining a large belly. Our culture is shown through advertising that having a flat belly is our goal in fitness. Many people think the core is about strong abs, but the core is not just abs, but strengthening the back muscles as well. If your goal is to have rock hard abs, then you are doing yourself a disservice because yoga teaches we have a second brain in our power center just above the navel, what you may know as chi energy, which is called Hara energy from my yoga training. There needs to be a balance of strong and softness in the belly to hear the body's wisdom. If you have ever done some abdominal crunches in the morning you would feel the power in your belly for the reminder of the day. The belly in yoga is where the third chakra resides. Chakra means wheel; it is what is known as spiritual anatomy in which we have wheels of energy spinning in certain areas around our body parts. The third center is the power source for all humans. I'm sure you have heard or said the phrase yourself, "I had a gut instinct about something." A medical doctor, Michael Gershon M.D. did a study on this center and is quoted as saying, "You have more nerve cells in the gut than you do in the combined remainder of the peripheral nervous system." He says he's quite sure that our thoughts and emotions are influenced by the gut.

The diaphragmatic, belly breath is important not just in golf. I have practiced it in playing badminton and basketball. Engaging the breath from your center gives more power to sports. I teach using this breath and energy of chi or hara while putting. Our putting stroke is shorter than a full out swing so we need a shorter breath. Inhale from the belly on the backstroke and exhale while following through the putt. It also aids in keeping the head down and eventually you can **will** the ball into the hole using this breath.

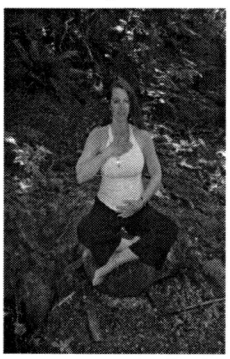

Complete breath

Moving on to the **Complete Breath** remember to breath through the nose.

Pia Nilsson must have taught a similar breath to Annika Sorensten. In Annika's book she describes playing with the men in the historical tournament and she related that "she was never so nervous at a first tee before, she described how she had to use deep breathing to help bring her to a calm and composed state."

It's best to start this breath off by imagining the lungs as having three parts- the lower (the belly breath), the middle (rib cage), and the upper (clavicle).

- Always begin this breath by exhaling the air completely.
- Begin inhaling starting with the lower lungs visualized and/or felt being filled first, then the middle and finally the upper. Pause for a second.
- Then exhaling, reverse the order, releasing first the upper lobes, then the middle and finally the lower, contracting the abdomen right back by imagining the belly button sinking back towards the spine.
- Pause again for one second with all the air expelled but don't tense up.

Try a couple of these breaths now in a continuous smooth movement. The inhalation is carried only to the point of fullness without strain. The exhale is a very important part of this breath; the slower the exhale the more relaxed one becomes.

I would encourage you to begin practicing before going to sleep at night. When you practice the complete breath in combination with the word reeelaaax, then you'll find by saying the relax all on it's own you don't have to consciously deepen your breath just watch and notice your breathing naturally increases of its own accord.

Whenever you have problems falling asleep, this little aid will have you falling off to dreamland in no time.

Easy Breathing –
Rhythmic breathing can be transferred into a rhythmic golf swing. If the top two breaths are hard to practice at first, simply try this pattern.
- **Breathe in to the count of four**
- **Breathe out to the count of eight, practice the full exhale by pulling your belly back towards the spine.**

Benefits of Deep Relaxed Breathing = Tempo and Timing
With Proper Deep Breathing you can,
- Hit pure powerful shots
- Overcome first tee jitters
- Become calm and composed
- Play to your full potential with longer, fluid, more rhythmic swings.

The Complete Breath combined with the Golf Swing

It was from my yoga training of breathing into the postures using the complete breath that I transferred the idea of using the Complete breathe with swinging the golf club. I had a miraculous experience immediately and I believe this is what hooked me on bringing this knowledge to golfers. I used it myself for a year before opening my yoga for golf business. All the findings were used my in own game before sharing with others.

YES! Yoga *Effortless* Swing

THE MOST IMPORTANT TOOL IN THIS WHOLE BOOK!!!

You will discover the secret of using the breath with the swing and witnessing more power behind your drives. First let me tell you that I can only bring you to it, I can't make you do it. The reason I say this is because in the early years my students would practice in class but not many would apply it to their game. I fixed that problem by adding one class at a driving range. This increased the success rate. I found junior golfers to be the most receptive in integrating this lesson of breathing with the swing and I was even told by some of them *"don't tell anyone else about this."*

A testimonial from a CPGA Golf Pro on the practice of one swing thought and using the Complete Breath with the swing.

"This is like magic HOW come no one knows about it?"
- Darryl Bailey

Begin by practicing the Complete Breath at the Driving Range first helps bring confidence before adding this new routine to your games.

Let's begin by imagining we are at the driving range, first you watch me and see how *effortless* my drives are. I explain this is what is known as the Yoga *Effortless* Swing.

This involves first using one swing thought to replace all the instructions and over time that can one swing thought can also be dropped and just the complete breath alone will be sufficient. I like to start golfers out with the word RELAX because the body will do as you command. You will notice the hands soften, the jaw and shoulders all let go naturally with this one word. Other words that can be used are FREEDOM, RELEASE, or RHTHYM.

Each word is broken down into long syllables for example using the word relax, begin with the inhale mentally say, <u>reeee</u> and with the exhale say <u>laxxx</u>. As a pre-shot routine- Take two complete breaths saying in your mind reelaxx as instructed above. Then simultaneously the swing is combined with your chosen word and Complete Breath. Sounds complicated in the written form but it is quite easy when practicing physically. Without stopping the next breath in, say reee with the back swing and exhale laax with the follow through swing. (Remember each exhale is longer than the inhale use your navel as a guide by drawing it in towards the spine. This way the inhale deepens naturally all on its own)

If I am really nervous I will not take a practice swing first I will take three breaths in set up and the fourth I will swing. Through experimenting I found that even though it seems like a long time to address the ball it is not. If I make a drive when I am still nervous I do not get the consistent straight drives and I spend more time on the fairway, either looking for my ball or playing from bad lies for the next shot. I now will take one extra breath and I am always rewarded with a great shot!

The longer the breath the longer the drives, this builds over time as the lungs develop.

Deep, rhythmic breathing is a useful tool to clear your mind and emotions to bring you back to a focused moment and put things into perspective. From the calm places we remember why we are out on the golf course; to have fun, meet new people, challenge ourselves in healthy ways, and enjoy the scenery and connect to Mother Nature. It is also one way to break the habit of always focusing on mechanics, and to balance the conscious mind and the sub-conscious mind to work together in harmony. We are here to allow the life principle to flow through us rhythmically and harmoniously.

To reiterate the belly breathing is associated with the putting stroke, and the Complete Breath with driving the ball. Chipping could fall in between these two breaths, depending on the amount of swing you must take for the shot before you.

"It's been a while since I've contacted you, and I wanted you to know how much I appreciated your help with the whole yoga for golf concept. Last year I was eliminated in the first round of match play at our club (28 handicap). This year my handicap dropped to 21. I just won the C flight match play championship, and my wife Barb and I won the couples match play, the final match with my 81. Most of the credit goes to the mental game. What a difference! Next year: B flight!"

Thanksagain!
Blair Hammond

The next breath Kapalabhati or **Breath of Fire** is the most outstanding beneficial cleansing breath in all of Yoga. It is not done while playing but at home sitting with a nice straight spine.

Kapalbhati Breathing:
Discover a Powerful Mind Detox Technique
                    To Bring The 'Spark' Into Your Life

A powerful breathing technique that is proven to help overcome blues, negativity, stress and depression - in a minute! This simple breathing exercise is known for its tremendous healing capability and ability to optimize your health and well-being.

It is the only technique used exclusively for mind purification among all the Yoga cleansing routines.

Precaution- Do not perform this breath during menstruation, as it creates internal heat and you want to keep the body cool at this time of the month.

Instructions:
- Relax your stomach muscles.
- Now expel the air as forcefully as you are comfortable with through the nose.
- This should cause the abdominal muscles to contract sharply and should draw
- the abdomen inwards towards the spine (like when you suck in your stomach). Then allow the inhalation to occur completely passive ly without any additional effort. To repeat, the exhalation is done using conscious sharp force, while the inhalation is just a recoil action bringing the air back into the lungs. All the breathing takes place through the nose. Right after the passive inhalation, exhale again forcefully and continue at a steady rhythm.
- Do a round of 10 exhales.
- Work your way up to doing 5 rounds, while taking a break between each round.

Benefits-
Practiced over time, Kapalbhati Pranayama also helps reduce abdominal fat, fight obesity, tone abdominal muscles and bestow core abdominal strength and power.
- **From an emotional stand point** -Kapalbhati Pranayama purges the system of accumulated emotional debris such as anger, hurt, jealousy,

hatred etc., thus dissolving the blockages
- **From a mental stand point**- Kapalbhati Pranayama assists in throwing out all negative thoughts from the psyche thus, helping to cleanse and illuminate the mind.
- **From a body stand point** -Kapalbhati Pranayama should be used to eject any illnesses, diseases, weaknesses from the body thus allowing it grow in health, vitality and vigor.

Secondary:
- Generates heat in the system to help dissolve toxins and waste matter.
- Adds luster and beauty to your face.
- Increases focus and concentration is multiplied, children can even use this if they have a hard time concentrating in school.

Cooling Breath - Sitali Breath (Sitali means cold)
- First we learn this sitting down until we feel confident to walk and breathe this breath at the same time.
- Sit with spine straight and erect.
- Open your mouth slightly and curl your tongue on to the roof of your mouth.
- Inhale a slow breath through the sides of your tongue making the noise like sucking up a straw.
- Close your mouth and relax your tongue - Hold your breath for the count of 5.
- Then exhale slowly through your nose.
- Repeat five times while learning, and as many as you need when you are overheated on the golf course.

Benefits-
- Cools the system and purifies the blood
- Calms the mind and nervous system
- Relieves thirst
- Stimulates liver and spleen
- Reported to help lower fevers

The last Major PGA Tournament of 2007 was played at Southern Hills in Okalahoma and temperatures reached over one hundred degrees. The players had a hard time and many were practicing at 4:00 oclock in the morning to avoid the heat. If you are ever in a similar situation playing in a heat wave, one pranayama that has been a lifesaver is the Sitali Breath or cooling breath, because when we are hot and bothered it's hard to be in the mood for all the positive upbeat thinking. It's hard to be in the moment. Frustration can set in quickly for yourself or your playing partners. When you get this breath down, then you can pass it on to your partner, unless of course it's a tournament and you want the edge. Think of this breath as the coolant for your engine that helps you from overheating.

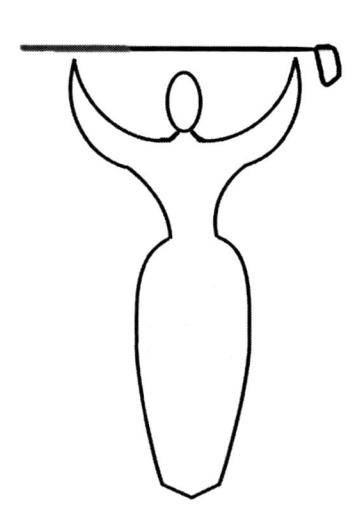

Come, Be Golfing Goddesses!

Goddess Isis representing the Back Nine

Hole 11 - Relaxation

Let us learn to relax into the lap of Isis the Great Mother and view her as a loving mother who protects and guides us. The mother figure of Isis can help us return to our own natural rhythms and the rhythm of mother earth.

"You don't play golf to relax you have to be relaxed to play golf."
- George Knudson

When I do a workshop on *Powerful drives, Powerful lives*, I ask the women what power means to them. The answers vary from being in control to surrendering control to a higher force. Think about what power means to you! In the practice of yoga the principle of surrendering equals being relaxed, hence you gain more power. This is just one of the many paradoxes in golf and it has been the hardest concept for many male students I have taught. Softness translates as Power. To transfer this on the golf course is an excellent way in both mind and body. Let's just talk about the power of the body right now. The more relaxed you are the more powerful drive you have. I'm sure you have either experienced this or seen it in someone else. When you try to kill the ball the result is a dribble. When you are at the driving range, with no pressure, the ball usually goes longer and farther. Add the pressure of the first tee and all those great drives at the driving range seem to be all played out. Tension is the enemy to any golf swing. What I usually find is that people are in a perpetual state of tension and don't really know how to relax at will. This is one of the reasons we begin at home to prepare ourselves before we even arrive at a golf course. The website has a place to sign in for your free MP3 on progressive relaxation this is an excellent tool to help retrain the body to come back its natural state of being. *www.golfinggoddesses.com*

Most of us know what tension feels like, but now we want to have the feeling of relaxation to be deeply imbedded. Begin to listen to this segment everyday and you will find more power in all areas of your life with this one simple act. Why? Because you will be removing blocked energy and letting a new energy move through you effortlessly. Just notice how others start responding to you differently and commenting on your subtle change before you even recognize it.

The mp3 will also help you integrate what you learned in the last chapter, combining the complete breath with the golf swing, as well as mentally saying reee-laaax, and to notice how different parts of the body begin to let go. In your set up you will soon notice the grip slightly softens and the jaw relaxes noticeably. If you ever had a golf pro tell you to relax your grip you can be relieved to know you don't have to go through a long process of breaking this habit of clenching. Just say Relax in place of instructions. Since we are trying to eliminate more commands to our already maxed out minds by saying "relax" it happens naturally and the less we think about it the better. We allow our body to make a smooth unencumbered shot. And remember a secondary occurrence of using the one swing shot with the breath, the deeper the breath the more oxygen is brought to the cells, which allows the muscles to *lengthen and elongate*. With the muscles lengthened come longer drives!

Relaxation is also the first ingredient to training the mind, one very powerful tool at your disposal is visualization. The easiest way to have consistency is to use visualization. What you form in your imagination is as real as any part of your body.

The idea, goal and the thought are real and will one day appear in the outside, material world if you are faithful to your mental image. AS WITHIN, SO WITHOUT, The outside mirrors the inside. External action follows internal action.

Today scientists explain the neurons that fire in our head are the same whether we imagine something or do it, if we watch something then close our eyes and remembered what we just watched. The imagery and the visual light up the same area in the brain. You will discover more evidence of this truth throughout the book.

Begin as soon as you can to say "I am a Great Golfer" and one day you will have more and more wins. One of the best ways to practice this is in a relaxed state, remember all the perfect hits you have made. YOU HAVE MADE amazing shots with your woods, your irons, and with your putters. Know that your muscles remember how to do this, your muscles remember how to play well. The more you visualize this, and feel the good feelings of great shots, the faster the good shots will come to the material plane. The best part about this inner preparation is that it doesn't take any extra time, the best time is just as you are drifting off to sleep at night or before rising in the morning. When the body is totally relaxed the powers to attract what you desire, is multiplied. It is scientific fact that the mind can't tell the difference between what is done physically or mentally.

I would use this example for my students, "Think about going to see a sad movie, your literal thinking mind knows that you are only seeing lights projected by the screen. But the characters have you so involved emotionally that your body responds by crying. It is not real what you are watching but the body is only reacting to the images from the mind."

Another story I always refer to when I am teaching, maybe you have heard of it. Is the war prisoner who imagined playing golf everyday to keep his sanity and hope. I believe this practice also kept him alive as he did not sink into despair and give up.

The wonderful results was when he played a golf game just after his release; when he was still weak and suffered from malnutrition, he played better then ever and actually took 20 strokes off his game and shot a 74! There are two book resources I found this story in:

•Second Edition of - Chicken Soup for the Soul
The Psychology of Winning- by Dennis Whitely

Now if you have never experienced the relaxation of a yoga class, I want to share with you what was written by a reporter who came to a beginner session. I hope it will inspire more women to try a gentle yoga class to feel the effects of true relaxation.

At the end of each yoga class we would have a relaxation time I would say to the class, "Breathe in the Extraordinary and Breathe out the Ordinary."

So Sheila titled the article Breathe in Extraordinary.

Breathe in Extraordinary

Written by Sheila Duncan

Yoga always sounded kind of hokey and somewhat mystical...until I tried it.

Now I am starting to truly appreciate it. Okay, so the stretching and exercise component is probably good for me, but what I really like is the concentration on breathing (something I would never take the time to do in a normal harried day) and the relaxation and release of tension (something I am not good at but am willing to learn).

Like most people, I usually rush to those sessions and 90 minutes later I am literally falling asleep.

Now that's therapy.

In the picturesque surroundings of Mono Centre, instructor Peggy Brigham tells us to breathe out the stress we experienced already in our day and let our minds wander as we make time for us. Like many people I have trouble getting my mind, body and spirit together any day of the week. But through yoga I am getting closer to that goal.

We're told not to feel guilty about taking time for us – and that is something women need to practice. We are usually running from one thing to the next and when we aren't our minds are.

The simplicity of it all is what appeals. We get to slow down and actually listen to our bodies breathe.

As we try out different poses and stretches, breathing techniques and relaxation tips we really are being taught flexibility and focus.

I love the feeling of being centered and actually focusing on my breathing. Not many people I know fit that into their day. But they probably should.

Peggy says yoga is more than stretching- "it's mastering a state of mind". Well my state is usually scattered, overloaded and overwhelmed. So noting and appreciating

my breathing is a minor miracle. The breathing seems to calm the mind and emotions.

Peggy says she was first introduced to yoga by her mother. "it made her calm and she made me a believer. When I became stressed I would get the yoga book and start on

my own." Yoga, she says, changed her attitude, making her more relaxed and accepting.

I think we could all handle some of that.

"You 'go with the flow' in yoga. It sounds pretty good to me. "Your mind is focused, your body is relaxed and fit, and that gives you flexibility."

We never make the time to have a focused mind.

Peggy has been teaching yoga since 1997. According to Peggy, most people like the relaxation aspect, the releasing of stress.

Her sessions start off with people selecting an angel card and a heart card from her basket. They are positive words or phrases of affirmation. "It helps centre you. We come in and our minds are full of chatter. The world can be harsh but this is nurturing. Yoga is about the whole being, not just he physical. And it is indeed nurturing. Where else would we hug our legs and feet and rock them like babies. Where else would we learn about breath control and try different breaths like the breath of joy and the alternate nostril breath for clarity of mind (not to mention getting rid of headaches).

"The internal organs are being massaged and cleansed," Peggy says, in reference to the poses that get us more in tune with our bodies.

The spirit gets massaged too.

And that helps you on the path to self-realization, wherever that is.

"It's very subtle," she says, adding that some people go to yoga to relax and they find themselves opening up to new ideas. It all depends on attitude.

Yoga has been around for thousands of years, shows you how to listen to your body and is not competitive.

And as Peggy says, it is a nice time out. It reinforces the message that we are worth it. "It works," she says.

Anything that can get me "in the flow, in the moment, has me so relaxed I am listening to my breathing and controlling it, and makes me feel good has a high value. Being in sync is the right place to be in all that we do.

Don't worry, I won't be striking any funny yoga poses the next time you see me but I do always look forward to the next class.

Peggy ends each session by saying "namaste" to the class. It means "the divine in me recognizes the divine in you".

Respectful, affirming, healthy…it doesn't get much better than that.

The View from Here/ 2001- Sheila Duncan
Reprinted with permission from The Citizen Newspaper

Prayer to Isis –
*Please give us the power to relax in our
pursuit of progress versus perfection.
So Mote it Be.*

Part 2
Direction South - Element Fire

Goddesses of Fire-
Pele a Hawaiian Goddess &
Kali a Hindu Goddess

- *Season: Summer*
- *Ceremony- Summer Solstice*
- *Quadrant of Day –Midday*
- *Stage of Life-Adolescent*
- *Color and Race- Red*
- *Represents the Heart/Spirit*

Qualities of Fire- The magic of creation involve learning to use the deaths within your life as opportunities for rebirth. Fire is destructive as well as creative.

Powers of the South- Passion, inspiration, creativity and fire in the belly

SOUTH - Fire - Passion

Growth in the South is the time of Summer. From the bloom we transform into the fruit of the labors. It is the time of mid-day, the hottest part of the day, the part when the sun is overhead and no shadows are cast.. Maturing and growing into an adult to be that we are. It is the time to accept the change and learn, to understand. Red is for fire, passion, time of fertility. The South is the place of passion in all things, sex, fertility, mating - the fires that burn within. The direction of fire, like the phoenix we can rise from the flames, we take and rise again from childhood into being an adult in the direction of the South

Yoga poses for Fire– poses **182-187**
Golfers Sun Salutation, Sphinx, Cobra, Warrior 2, and Triangle

Chapter 3

Pele – Hawaiian Fire Goddess Passion and Freedom

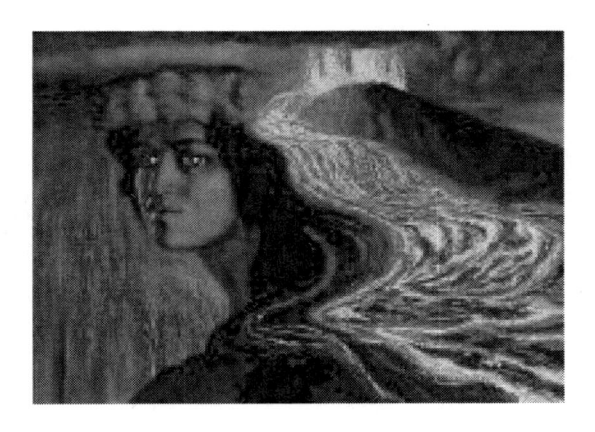

Myth - Pele is a fire Goddess of lightning, dance, volcanoes, and violence. Goddess Pele is like a normal human when it comes to feelings, but she is more of a Goddess when it comes to rage and anger. Even if she is the slightest bit annoyed, then she will start a volcanic eruption of some sort or a lava flow.

Goddess Pele was and still is famous for the different forms she can be and for the fiery rage she would go into when her temper got high. She is also famous for the different types of explosions she could be.

Goddess Pele is the Hawaiian Goddess of fire and volcanoes.
She is capable of both these objects.
-Wikipedia encyclopedia

Personal message: Pele's appearance signals a need for awakening. Have you been sitting still for too long? Have you been lulled into sleep by the evenness in your life?

Come, Be Golfing Goddesses!

Has reality been too slippery to grasp? Get ready to awaken your awareness and come into full consciousness. Now is the time to see things as they really are, to initiate change so things can be as you want them to be. Now is the time to wake up to your potential and power, to move and shake. Pay attention to all that life is telling you. The Goddess says that when you nurture awakening, your life becomes creative rather than reactive, an infinitely more powerful place to be!

http.www.angelfire.com/va/goddesses/pele/html

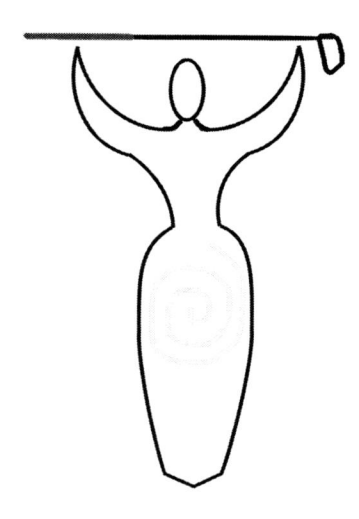

Goddess Pele representing the Front Nine

Hole 3 - Passion

By reading Pele's Myth and her personal message, she is telling us to wake up, allow yourself to get angry at injustices. Anger can be your friend, embrace that passionate
side of yourself, it can tell you if you are acting or doing something because others want you to. On some level, you do not want to act or do or be that way, so anger arises. Learning to assert ourselves and say no is better then being aggressive and out of control like a Goddess. My mother always told me "you can get more flies with honey then vinegar." Meaning people respond better if you are sweet instead of bitter in your approach.

We certainly want to be in control of our emotions on the golf course - it helps if we can view Golf Courses like our Mother - Our Mother Earth to all beings. I have been shown the Goddess is coming back in subtle ways.

If you decide to research the Goddess path through the many sources out there, you will understand that what was sacred to the Goddess was turned around to look evil. The Language of the Goddess was made to be degraded. The word Bitch became a naughty word in Christian Europe, Barbara G. Walker tells us, "because it was one of the most sacred titles of the Goddess, Artemis-Diana, leader of the Scythian alani or 'hunting dogs'. The Bitch-goddess of antiquity was known in all Indo-European cultures, beginning with the Great Bitch Sarama who led the Vedic dogs of death."

I like the modern term for Bitch –
> **B**abe
> **I**n
> **T**otal
> **C**ontrol
> of
> **H**erself.

As women we have been conditioned not to be the bitch, to be givers and be kind. Let's use the golf course to remember who we are. We can emulate a Babe in total control of herself by walking proudly to every shot instead of emulating a lot of men and their displacement of anger. I have seen a few women act out in temper - taking the game way too seriously, playing golf like many men. Men and advertising think it is okay to display temper tantrums on the course and throw their clubs. But Ladies, let us be more mature than that! We want to view the golf course as a sacred place where we are playing a game between our higher selves and our egos. Golf is a spiritual game. Just look at the many spiritual books that have come out since *Michael Murphy's 'Golf and the Kingdom,'* which tells the tale of Shiva Irons and his mystical teachings. It makes for an unpleasant game for others when one person can't control their temper. Men knew this once, when golf was called a Gentlemen's game, and we can bring them back to it by playing in a new sacred way ourselves. A game that has more soul, more substance, that can help us on our spiritual paths.

The dictionary interpretation of the word Gentle is: *kind and amiable, mild and refined in manner, quiet and sensitive of disposition, meek and moderate, of good family.*

Our society tells us it is a weak person who has traits of being kind, amiable, mild and refined in manner. But I assure you all these qualities take strength to acquire and to live and golf by. Who would you rather play golf with - someone who is quiet, cultured and relaxed, or a sour, obnoxious golfer? It is easy to give in to anger and frustration. Maybe these golfers need to see more examples of calm and composed golfers to realize it is possible to play consistent rounds of golf in a fun and enjoyable way.

Passion reignited -Setting Goals
One way to gain control over our emotions and make golf fun is by setting Goals and using our imaginations. Look at life - without a purpose, a vision or goal, we tend to drift aimlessly and stay in victim consciousness. The same with golf, we can drift aimlessly throughout the golf season and letting life surprise us, or we can get clear on what we want and begin to co-create it with the magic of mother earth.

To begin to co-create any area of your life it doesn't matter how insignificant happens when you understand that there is always a partnership going on. To begin to recognize this partnership is when we use the spiritual way of setting goals. It starts by focusing on our desires and than the next important next step is releasing them and not to get stuck in thinking about how or when they arrive. When we have passion and desire and then let go of the outcome we are on our way to learning the higher lessons of becoming a Creatrix. This then leads to a more passionate life as we let the Goddess lead the way.

I like to ask my students what excites them about the game of golf? Just as instructed with affirmations the more good feelings we engage in our goal setting, the quicker they will appear. Have you ever had a hole-in-one? Have you thought seriously about achieving this? Think about how happy and excited you would be if you got a hole in one? Let us begin to focus on the dreams of golf, not the problems. Let's bring imagination, passion and excitement to our games. Fun enhances everything, Fun ... enhances golf, fun enhances life and fun enhances yoga.

Goals give us direction and purpose. Goals are fun they generate interest and enthusiasm in golf and life. They make your game more challenging. Desire when harnessed is Power.

"Surrender to desire and gain energy, enthusiasm, mental zip and even better health. Energy increases, multiplies, when you set a desired goal and resolve to work toward that goal. There is magic in setting and writing down goals. It sets up into motion a powerful psychological, spiritual and emotional force. We become aware of the things we need to do, to achieve and accomplish them. Things come to us, things begin to happen. We tap into our powerful subconscious mind."

- David Schwartz, The Magic of Thinking Big.

Goals help us to have more control and direction. The biggest paradox is you never really have control unless you surrender to a higher consciousness. You can create your golf game and create your life but only in partnership with the ultimate Creator/Creatrix.

So we set goals, whether it is as simple as playing more golf in a season, to breaking 100, 90, or even getting a hole in one. But let's take for example getting a hole in one. You set the goal, then let go of the outcome. It may come in the first year you set it or maybe in the following years. It mainly falls into the category of your self-discipline. The more disciplined you are with your intention and focus the faster you will achieve the results. The steps require writing down the goals, saying them over and over, and seeing and feeling yourself as already achieved the goal.

Let us go deeper into this. These steps are the same as in any self-help book. Write down the goals and visualize them as already completed in as much detail as possible. It is best to begin with small reachable goals. Success breeds success. It is far better to make reasonable, reachable ideals, which allow you to enjoy success, instead of high ideals which may be a way of setting yourself up for fear and disappointment. Then when you truly feel good and successful about yourself, you can set new higher attainable goals. This is one way to insure victory by improving your game slowly step by step. What we are after is genuine lasting improvement instead of drifting through each golf season with no vision or wanting instant gratification. Remember this way of playing is a journey, one golf season at a time.

The key to bringing your goal into reality starts first as a thought form. The secrets of the Far East can be summed up in one word - belief. How do the yogis walk across fire without burning their feet? Belief they can do it. Mind over Matter. They spend time in meditation, visualizing themselves with the feat already accomplished with no burns. This is how I have accomplished my goals in life and my golf games in my head by seeing yourself already doing it and it has worked for others. Think of the mental process involved in taking a trip.

Have you ever stopped to analyze the process involved? First you get the idea for the trip. Then you decided where you would go. Shortly after you began to visualize yourself packing for the trip, making all the arrangements, meanwhile you focus the most on the fun part, shopping, relaxing on the beach, playing a golf course, going out for meals. The vacation turned out because you saw yourself doing it before it became a reality. You clearly put yourself in the picture. There was an expenditure of energy and most of it came naturally to use our imaginations before you actually experienced it in material form.

In other words it is not only necessary to feel and think yourself successful, it is important to go one step further and actually see yourself as already having arrived in the performance of your goal. The next step is to stay open to your gut feelings, your instincts while playing and to keep your logical mind out of the way. If you have promptings to use a different club, then go with the first thought. Have faith and belief in your sub-conscious mind to carry out your sincerest hopes and desires this takes practice but over time it adds passion and excitement to all your games.

I would like to add that there is another element in setting goals and that is the courage to follow the signposts that come our way. Many times we may be presented by an opportunity that looks like a problem in disguise. I will share one such opportunity that I did not follow through on, when I lived in Ontario. I lacked the courage, yes, but also my ego got in the way.

In the small town where I lived in, there was an annual Million dollar Hole - in - One contest that any one could participate in which went from Thursday to Sunday. Now on Sunday the cut off time to qualify was in the morning and then the afternoon was for all the participants who had gotten closest to the hole or had a hole-in-one on any of the given days leading up to cut off time. If you did have a hole-in-one it did not count for the million dollars, it just qualified you for Sunday afternoon.

At the time I was writing a bi-weekly column in the sports section of a local paper in which I gave tips to golfers. I decided to write an article about steps for training the mind to win the million dollar hole-in-one – the article came out a month before the event was scheduled.

This is what I wrote and I began personally to put my words into practice.

'Mental Training for the Million Dollar hole-in–one - if this is one of your goals you must begin the mental practice NOW! To accomplish this or any goal you must have a strong desire. Desire is the key. Wishful thinking will not bring it about, since the negative self-talk can easily sway you into thinking it will never happen. It takes discipline to outtalk your negative thoughts, which may sound something like this "it would be nice to win, but it is impossible." "I'm here to tell you nothing is impossible. As Henry Ford said "Whether you think you can or you think you can't, you're right." The process involves seeing yourself in your set up position, swinging the club and seeing the ball going into the hole. Since it is only a few weeks away, this has to be practiced over and over again with relaxed concentration to effectively train the mind.

Now you may say, "I don't have any extra time to do this." Well, it doesn't take any extra time; the best time to practice is just as you are falling asleep at night and as you are waking up in the morning. Practice over and over ... sounds simple - right? Wrong, the inner dialogue that is always judging and evaluating will pipe up with some thoughts to get you to stop. Don't give into these thoughts. That's all they are, just thoughts and you don't have give them any power. Pretend you can place them in a garbage can with a lid on them. In my research on mental training I came across interview with a talk show host named Dini Petty. She asked the man in the Guinness Book of Records (at the time) for the most holes-in-one (he had 15) what his secret was. His answer was that he visualized his shot going in every time. By practicing this inner game routine of visualizing the ball going in he provided a vision or plan for his muscles to follow."

Following my own advice, I was very impressed with how close each ball was going directly to the target. In my set up position, I gave myself the command "In the Hole". I didn't think another thought, I just let my body respond to this command. I only went one day that year, but I was excited that I had evidence this will work. Each ball I drove went exactly where I envisioned and sooo close. I had participated the previous years without any mental training and did not come as close to the target as I did that year. I thought to myself, " I will do it for sure next year because I will start practicing the inner work months ahead not weeks". In hindsight I think to myself "how much passion did I really have; I was only experimenting with walking my talk. In hindsight I realize that it went deeper than that, I believe I sabotaged myself with "the fear of success". My inner thoughts said "Did I really deserve the million dollars?" So through this goal I learned about my deeper hidden belief.

    In 2006 I did in fact start my visualization of seeing the ball go in the hole before I went to bed at night. I have learned when I am in a relaxed state that my subconscious mind doesn't distinguish if it was a real experience or not. I began the process in December in February I met a man who had a booth across from mine at a health show. He was looking at my portfolio and saw my article on the million-dollar-hole in one and said this spring he was starting up a tour of the million- dollar- hole in one to go to different locations. I thought, "Wow! This is great.

    Through my visualizations the law of attraction has brought us together and now I will have many opportunities not just in my hometown." Well one part of me wanted success but the sabotaging self was stronger. I lost his card. No matter, I still believed that I would win in my hometown. So I kept visualizing, but another goal that I had for many more years began to take form and become a reality, which was when my kids were grown, I was going to travel and specifically live in B.C. I had been talking about it for years and with more intent the last couple of years. My friend, who was out here, was even scouting out jobs for me. So what happened? Well we left before schedule. Luckily we were open to the flow and it all happened effortlessly until we actually got on the road. We were pulling our trailer and just as we got to Muskoka our transmission gave us some warning signs. We ended up making it to my cousin's place and, after checking out prices, it was cheaper to go back to Toronto where I purchased the car for a new trany. Well we had to wait until he had the time and could get one. It just so happened we went back on the same weekend that Orangeville had its million-dollar-hole-in–one. I thought, "this is interesting; maybe I can still enter", but the shop didn't have any cars on loan at the moment.

    I was staying at my brother's, an hour away from Orangeville, so I surrendered. I knew it wasn't going to happen. But then things were taking longer with the parts. He said he could get me a car for Sunday. That would have been so perfect; the Universe had set it all up through the inconvenience of having to go back and what did I do - I missed out on the opportunity. I said, "No, I don't need the car." My ego voice piped up with thoughts saying things like, "You can't go back to Orangeville everyone thinks you are gone already." Or "It will be a waste of time." you get the point. My fear stopped me, fear of what, success maybe? So now I am in a province where a million dollars is nothing. Because of living in a small town I thought a million was like a billion. Now I have expanded my reality. There are apartment condos here selling for a million. Unheard of. I live 10 minutes away from West Vancouver now and million dollar homes are the starting price for many of them.

Now I am convinced, one million dollars is not asking for much. I have taken a good look at my belief system so I can thank this part of me that has been protecting me from having lots of money for some reason. I believe it is because my line of work, teaching yoga, and the spiritual teachings, that holds a discrepancy inside me. I am working on bridging the East and the West inside of me when it comes to green money energy. My opportunity for a hole-in-one will just have to come on a golf course. There is still no reason why I should stop visualizing myself doing it.

When teaching this theme to my class I give them a piece of paper and ask them to write out their goals while there, so I am assured they do it. I don't need to see the goal but I stress how important it is to write it down for their sub-conscious mind to start the process of bringing what they want to them. I like to ask then how many people put down as a goal to get a hole- in- one. Not many do; they don't think it's possible, but why not? Isn't this the whole goal in golf?

To get the ball in the hole in the least shots possible, so it stands to reason that every par three on the course is a potential waiting to happen, only most golfers don't view it that way, or they may have at the beginning of learning the game but then it is usually par they want to make.

The biggest challenge is trusting, letting go of expectations, of the past, future and live in the present moment of each shot. Let go of each shot good or bad and move on. In the movie Tin Cup with Kevin Costner, who plays a golf pro, he says to a woman who is taking a lesson, "Golf is all about gaining control of your life and letting go at the same time." We have learned that we can gain control by training our minds and then we let go by relaxing.

Come, Be Golfing Goddesses!

Goddess Pele representing the Back Nine

Hole 12 - Freedom

    I find it easier now to be unattached to the outcome of a day of golf compared to my earlier days of playing. I love the freedom! I now recognize if I have not practiced throughout the winter, and this could include indoor driving ranges as well as mental training, I should not have any expectations that I will be at the same level of play I was in the fall of the previous year. I used to be attached to my swing being the same in the spring as it was in the fall when I finished for the season and I would get very frustrated. With a lot of practice and understanding I have learned to accept how I swing the club each time I play and that was by consciously playing acceptance rounds of golf games. To me acceptance and freedom go hand and hand. With a mind-set of acceptance I have developed myself into a life long student my own natural rhythm as being my teacher and then I live the life of effortlessness. Every time I am impatient I know that is my ego thinking and when I release my expectations of the timing I am always shown the right way, one step at a time. This philosophy I apply to every single area of my life which any person can do to achieve freedom.

    I learned to live in the beginner mind every time I approached the game because of the philosophy of yoga. The importance of learning to let go and not be attached on the golf course really helped me in life. I could transfer this principle easier and I learned to understand the wisdom of the spiritual teachers who would tell students "Learn to let go, not be attached to any person, place or thing." You may, like me discover that this is a life long goal. It definitely helps to look at this attachment and nonattachment as a circular learning experience. Two steps forward, one step back. On some occasions it is easier than others. I believe compassion for ourselves when we slip back into being attached to the outcome is the best way to move forward again.

    I would like to share a story I heard from a man who did a talk on the subject of letting go. He used a description on how to catch a monkey. He related that if we were to go to the jungle with a large jar with a small opening at the top and put a banana in it we would catch a monkey.

    Since Monkey's have been caught this way before after their behavior had been observed. You see the monkey would put his hand in the jar and not be able to take the banana out. The monkey would be so attached to the banana it would actually drag the jar around which kept the monkey from climbing a tree. Which being the case would make it easy to catch. All the monkey had to do from not being caught was to let go of the banana and he would have been free of the jar. But he couldn't, he was too attached to the banana.

Now we think we are more intelligent then animals but some days I beg to differ.

We can get caught because we can't let go of our attachments, whatever they may be. That is what brings the suffering. It is very difficult at first to become the observer and just watch the thoughts and feelings and not become attached to them. An ancient description of the mind is relating it to a monkey's chatter. The lesson of the attached monkey can be used when we are first beginning meditations. The Father of Yoga Patanjali's tells us in his experience, "yoga is the breaking of contact with pain."

To the yoga tradition the pain is being stuck in Maya, Maya means the illusion. To explain how this tradition explains illusion would take another book. To simplify things let us think in the terms that with awareness we can break the pain. If we remember that yoga is a system that was designed to bring us to our higher selves we learn what part of us is acting from the ego and trying to control or are we operating from our higher self that is connected to our natural flow as we release pain from our bodies we also remove it from the Earth.

The promise of freedom is living with the awareness that life is impermanent. If we can accept the truth that life and death are partners. That there is a flow to life like the ocean tide, things come and they go. Just watch and you will notice there is a cycle of energy that moves things to us and away from us. This does not mean we are good or bad it is just a natural law as we accept this law we can begin to release many degrees of fear that are operating in the world. The ego is the mind that grasps, that clings like the monkey. Most people want the world in a certain way so they'll feel okay. When both my parents became sick at the same time before they passed on, my mantra was "it's not good or bad, it just is." My suffering came when I placed my own judgment on the situation. I watched how I was not responding to their needs I was reacting from a place of panic. In my release of judgment through this affirmation I regained my composure and was more loving and helpful in the process.

I may not have liked the situation but with acceptance I came out of the denial and felt a measure of peace with their death being the cycle they were in. So it wasn't my running around in a panic that got me the peace, it was the awareness. The awareness that has been handed down from the yogic teachings, "Do an action and let go of the outcome" and especially do it with the intent to offer your action to the higher dimension, whether you call that energy God/Goddess/ Universe or by any other name. The words don't matter as much as the intention.

The personalities we have developed are our egos. It is through the ego that most people play out their games and lives. The ego that has been bred in the western society has been to be aggressive, competitive, to achieve and constantly strive. It is very strong and it does not want to die. Because the ego is a part of every human there are different solutions to overcoming the ego to live more from our higher selves. In yoga the story of the battle between living in the ego self and living from the Higher self is told in The Bhagavad Gita. The same story is told in a different way in JRR Tolkens Lord of the Ring series in the last book 'The Return of The King.'

> *One should raise oneself by the Self, one should not degrade oneself.*
> *For the Self alone is the friend of the self.*
> *And the self alone is the enemy of the Self.*
> -Bhagavad Gita

I have always thought the book, *"The Legend of Bagger Vance"* by Stephen Pressfield is a brilliant transfer of Hindu's Holy book The Bhagavad-Gita and how it has been transposed into a golf game. In the truest sense we are playing a game between our ego, the small self, and our Higher Self.

The ego does serve a purpose but not as the master it believes itself to be. It needs to be retrained once again to follow the instructions of the heart and the hero within since we all have a blueprint inside that is uniquely ours. As we grow towards wholeness we must begin to trust our souls or big Self and begin to drop the personality that was formed by all the conditions of our culture, the media being the most relevant. I ask my students to take regular negativity diets, cut out or cut back for sometime each month from TV., radio, newspapers and even people in their lives whose habits are to report the doom and gloom of the world or their own world at the very least. We create our own world by our thoughts and images. We can make our life a living hell or heaven, we always have a choice.

This is the era to let go into the Great Mystery that has a perfect plan for each of us. Some people, who are in resistance with the natural rhythm and their own true self, do get the proverbial two- by- four across the head as a wake up call. Others are not so lucky and are suffering. But are they suffering with awareness, or because of brainwashing and habits? The masters have pointed out over and over again that this is a Free Will Universe, here's one more way of saying it

"Within each of us lies the power of our consent to health, and to sickness, to riches and to poverty, to freedom and to slavery. It is we who control these, and not another

- Richard Bach.

Prayer to Pele- Please bring us to our passion and help us let go of all resistance to the new. - so be it.

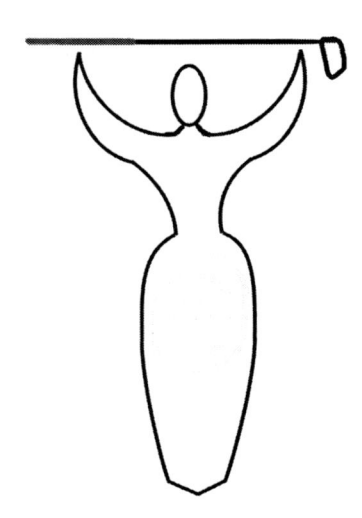

Chapter 4

Kali – Hindu Fire Goddess Patience and Persistence

Qualities – Kali is a Triple Goddess (Birth, Destruction, Resurrection)

Kali, the Dark Mother of India, embodies the most fearsome aspect of the Devi, the triple goddess symbolically represented by Parvati, Durga and Kali, maid, mother and crone (or my version princess, queen and wise woman). Although fearsome in appearance, the image of Kali is rife with spiritual symbolism. Her necklace of human heads represents total knowledge and wisdom of humanity.

In her many hands she holds weapons representing ways of detachment from binding illusions. Kali's powers of creation, preservation and destruction are represented in the truths and inner fears that we must face in time of profound change. Her energy moves through the cosmos in powerful waves, destroying what is no longer viable and creating something new and wonderful out of the formless matter that constitutes chaos.

Prayer to Kali

Kali, let us call upon you to assist us in surrendering and destroying the old habits and patterns of living that threaten our self-growth and survival. Strip us bare of pretense, and grant us the courage to confront the deepest fears that rob us of real freedom. Transform us into powerful agents of healing change, for ourselves, and the world.

Goddess Kali representing the Front Nine

Hole 4 - Patience

For me Kali represents Patience with her (Birth, Destruction, Resurrection) attributes. In the last chapter we talked about our passion in the form of goals and then detaching from those goals. Now it would be nice if it only took one season for all our goals to come to fruition. Some do yes if they are small, but it seems the bigger the goal the longer it takes. So how do we wait - patiently or impatiently? If we are impatient while going through Kali's cycles of birth, death and rebirth, then we are in a sense beating ourselves up and blaming it on outside events. It's not what happens to us that makes us happy or miserable, it's how we respond. Carlo's Castaneda said, *"We can make ourselves miserable or happy; the amount of work is the same."* One of the easiest ways to go through a growth spurt in your life is to accept responsibility. If we are unhappy, say in our job, the Universe will give us signals and chances to leave on our own.

If we lack the courage to make the changes the first few times, then the signals become stronger and harder until we are in enough pain that we have to change. My friend used to say that, "if you don't want to change, wait for the pain." Yes, it can be painful to wait for the next step, the patience to wait when one phase of your life is completed and the waiting for the birth of the next has not come into full form *or* has not even revealed itself to us. Usually the pain comes from not having faith that the Universe, the Goddess wants you to be empty before you fill up again to something even better then before. So embrace the darkness in Kali, the patience to go through the cycles. Play more golf! Why? Because this is a great playing field to learn to become patient. I once read that the virtue of patience is begotten by being patient. "Well," I thought, "That's great, how do I do that?" I found the answer through playing golf, but there are other games such as Chess that we can learn the art of patience from. Think about the one thing all the touring pros who win, say? They tell the world, "they stayed patient, Very, very patient." They didn't let what was before them determine what the outcome of the game was going to be. They stayed relaxed and calm, which is a byproduct of being patient. If your eyes are showing you that you just made three bogeys and you really want to win club championship this year, relax and trust your intuition. This is being patient. Use the centering technique in chapter nine and repeat to yourself over and over the mantra, "this is my game". Even if it's not, the next game will be. Every game has within it an opportunity to learn something so if you do lose the game, please don't lose the lesson.

We can't always be on the losing cycle, just as we can't always be on the winning cycle. Because we are one with the cycles, we are part of nature, like the Goddess Kali and other Goddesses who represent the Triple Energy. Believe in yourself and your ability to score. Patience, instead of pushing, frees up a bundle of energy. Pushing is impatience. The need to control it makes one rigid and stiff.

Jack Nickolas said, *"A player who could keep their head on straight down the stretch in a major tournament was the one who was most likely to be standing after all the shots have been fired."* He was referring to the value of being patient, thinking with a clear head and, most important, staying emotionally and mentally composed. Jack stayed composed throughout his career. The proof of the wisdom of his words is in the record books. He remains golf's definite model for ultimate patience and composure.

We all see the effects of living in a fast-paced society where instant gratification is often the norm. When we want something, we want it now. This sense of urgency is certainly reflected in our approach to the game of golf. The line up these days on public golf courses is growing longer every year. The tolerance level is growing shorter every year. The coping tools in this book will help develop tolerance and patience.

There was a time in the 50's and 60's when women first took to driving a car, there was so much ridicule women received from men. They viewed us as bad drivers because we were new at it. Now in car commercials women are portrayed just as competent as men. When people are new to anything, as women are viewed in golf, it takes time for the acceptance to over come the impatience.

Over the years the number one complaint I hear from women is how to deal with feeling rushed by the foursome behind them. Can we ignore other golfer's impatience? We need to change the perspective that the ones behind us are in control. I guess my question today would be, "Is it only when a foursome of men are behind you or is it any foursome?" The tools in chapter nine on centering teach how to guard ourselves against outside distractions, such feeling rushed. When you begin to react to feeling rushed, you play sloppy, you end up taking more time, and it goes into a perpetual circle of impatience. Then you are working at golf, not playing anymore. Stop, get centered, ignore the distractions and get back to the joy of the moment. You are out in nature, not doing chores; enjoy yourself more by becoming and staying composed. Then you will notice the group behind just fades away naturally.

Being patient with myself is a way of loving myself. When first moving to B.C. we lived on the small island of Salt Spring for eight months then we moved to North Vancouver I wrote in my journals that I was quite tired and didn't know why. My energy was going through yet another adjustment. We just got settled in Salt Spring and then it was time to pack up and move again. I wondered how I will have the energy to even teach some classes in the weeks ahead. Then I counseled myself to become to patience with myself. One day I may have lots of energy and the next day nothing. The gift now is to allow the energy that is moving through me on a given day to have its own way. This way I am not beating myself up with thoughts like, "What's the matter with me, why can't I get anything done today?" I just have to be patient and trust that the body knows when to act and move and the energy will propel me forward when that time comes.

I have seen this happen over and over. I feel stuck. I don't know why I try and push instead of going with the flow and then it is revealed later why I had to sit tight on a particular day or two. But even with this knowledge I still have times when I want to know answers all the time. I forget to live in the mystery. We are not taught that here in the West - to live in the mystery. One can only hope with the new science of quantum physics the mystery will be an exciting place that people want to live in.

Now Kali is almost too powerful for the Western cultures that generally wait for the pain to get a wake up call. To willingly call upon her guidance to go into the darkness is not something that is even considered, nor even really supported because we have lost touch with nature. One of the signs the female life force has been guiding us is through gardening. Look at the popularity in gardening and the many lessons we gain through the analogy of a garden. Patience is definitely one of them. Do you remember planting seeds in school and the teacher putting the cups of soil on the windowsill and witnessing the growing process? The seed needs to be put in the darkness of the soil first before coming out into the light. Have you tried growing things from a seed state lately? It is a great exercise in gaining patience.

Another thing I would like to share is the resting period of the winter months and then the new growth in the spring. One of the most painful lessons in the garden is pruning. You have waited months to have your flowers bloom and then we are told to cut the bushes back. Remember when first learning about your garden and what is good for rose bushes and you learned about pruning. We look at a healthy bush and logically we think, "Why would we want to cut this back?" but we do it because the seasoned experts tell us that it will later produce more foliage and flowers. Even through the doubt we follow the advice, we learn delayed gratification by doing this and with patience we find out that the experts told the truth. We do have much healthier, beautiful bushes. With these results we find every year it gets easier to trim back and prune. It may seem like Kali's darkness and destruction are trying to keep us from moving ahead, from reaching our potential but I believe it is all part of growth and our own blooming.

Growth is the way in which we ourselves change, and the natural world around us. For we learn that life is a progression, a movement, which is forever renewing itself through cycles of birth, death and regeneration. None of these states could stand-alone they are interdependent.

I have read the word regeneration many times in Goddess books and did not truly understand the meaning until I came to B.C. I have now experienced first hand what it means by going into the old growth forests. Those giant beauties that got chopped down did not die. They have become the birth place of many other trees and bushes growing out the top of the stumps, this is regeneration in action.

Another popular analogy of patience has been passed to us from farming. Many people use the analogy of a farmer who plants his crops in early spring. The farmer knows enough not to go out in late spring and pull up the shoots to see how much they have grown. No, he knows that in the summer or fall he can expect his crops to bear fruit. When we were in harmony with Nature and not trying to dominate her, we were also in harmony with change, but some where in time permanence became the dominating theme. Look at the hardship the last generation had with lay-offs. It was once believed and supported that you could work at one job until you retired. There was security, but how much happiness and creativity went with that job security. We still search for the security, and that can make for a painful life especially when it comes to aging gracefully. In the old days the female archetype was the central religious figure. We observed in women what was also observed in nature - the unfolding of the life cycle: reproduction, death and rebirth.

We worshipped the reproductive organs of plants, animals and humans since that is where the life force dwells. We once learned by observing how we planted our dead just as we planted seeds energy is never completely destroyed. After a period of rest, the energy of the corpse or seed is returned in one form or another. From death comes life even if we do not acknowledge this process today. We once loved the earth and thought of the natural environment as holy so we did not ever consider her as a garbage dump or to selling pieces of her off to the highest bidder to do what they will. When women were the religious figures it was the crone, the wise woman, that every woman aspired to be not the youth of the teenager years.

When I first began teaching my Goddess yoga in 1999, I had a few wise women in the sessions that emulated growing old gracefully. Spirituality was becoming more common in everyone's consciousness and it seemed like a time for empowering the crone years. As I watched, the women I taught moved on into the next phase of their life empowered. I was excited about reaching the next stage myself. I felt like a pre-teen waiting to be a teenager. That growing seed has been squashed in most of our western culture who are influenced by the media. What seems prevalent now is denial about aging, which incidentally is the wording for all the abundance of creams on all the shelves.

They are called anti-aging, anything to look and feel young again. This is so sad Women I encourage you to wake up, to the fact that you are beautiful, and you are perfect. Yoga can bring out your youthful spirit and your inner radiance, one Yogini taught Yoga until she was 102. The quick fix doesn't have to win out every time. We can say no - enough of giving our power away to advertising, enough of giving our power away to impatient people. Enough of giving our power away, period. Think on this, the crone years, can be a blossoming of the wise woman a most powerful era for changing the world. All we need is courage to follow our inner Goddess and things will flow effortlessly, for our good and the good of our Mother Earth.

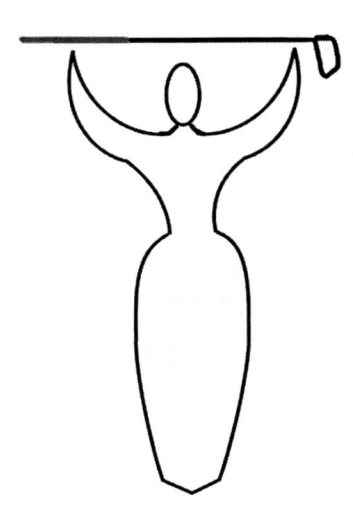

Goddess Kali representing the Back Nine

Hole 13 - Persistence

*Nothing in the world can take the place of perseverance.
Talent will not; nothing is more common than unsuccessful people with talent.
Genius will not; unrewarded genius is almost a proverb.
Persistence and determination alone are omnipotent.
The slogan, PRESS ON, has solved, and will always
Solve the problems of the human race."*

- Calvin Coolidge

    Do you need to learn golf for business and you just don't like the game? Do you want to learn the game but you can't seem to get any better. You've hit a plateau and you think why bother any more. Maybe it's not golf at all but there IS something in your life you feel frustrated about and you want to give it up? Or there is a persistent something that drives you? Maybe a creative talent you have, and are not utilizing? You say to yourself that you'll get to it one day when you have the time, or when the kids are grown, etc, etc. When all the excuses are out on the table, is there something that stills peeks out of the pile of papers? Is there some persistent force that wants to be noticed and acknowledged? What is this persistent energy? Could it be Kali's energy of creation that wants to be brought forth? I believe all women are creative since we have wombs, granted not all of our wombs are creating a human life, but it is still this center in our bodies which gives birth to projects, art, even lovemaking. Or maybe you are seeing that you have been in the process of living your ultimate gift to society and you are burdened with discouragement over and over again.

    It seems there is an obstacle to every success. Could this be Kali's energy of destruction? If you find yourself in the chaos, and you have thoughts of defeat, go play golf and learn from playing the game. Let us imagine the perfect, almost impossible desire, of a new golfer who never encounters an obstacle on the golf course. How would they know how to play well when one does come their way? Did you become discouraged when first learning the game and give up, or did you have the persistence to keep playing and become stronger and wiser after each obstacle. These obstacles are designed on purpose to make you lose your focus, to intimidate you, and challenge you, basically the hazards are just more head games. But it's through playing the game that we can build up resistance to the obstacles in other area of life, and through this experience, see life as a game as well. Obstacles are not really meant to break you, but make you. I believe in the statement that life only gives you what you can handle.

I learned a tip from a golf pro who told me, "after a particularly intimidating hole look back at it after it is all played out and you will see it from a different perspective." Once again the correlations to life, hindsight is 20/20 in golf and life. All we have to do is have the persistence to trust the Goddess that the path is a process and she has our highest interests at heart, even if we can't see it at the moment. If you can't get away to play golf, then the next best thing to do is yoga, be aware that yoga is a lifelong practice and that one develops a certain determination to show up on the mat, however they feel because we always feel better after.

Any worthwhile endeavor takes time, I encourage you don't give up before the rewards come. Again, as I mentioned under patience, delayed gratification is not taught in our society. I don't know if anyone has ever written about Tiger's persistence when he changed his swing but I have a great respect for him in the sense that he did not give in to the pressure of the media's negative bashing. He stayed true to his highest goal and did not give way to his ego. I went through a similar experience of changing my swing when he was changing his I was tempted many times to give into my ego, so he was a good role model for me. My ego was engaged already in the sense that I was practicing a new swing and I would leave my hometown and go to a distant driving range so I was less likely to see someone I knew. For you single girls, a driving range can be a great place to meet men. They always seem to want to help correct the swing and give their expert tips. I found that I really had to check my ego because with the new swing came new instructions so I wasn't hitting the ball very well. I was thinking of the mechanics. And when men came over to fix my stance or whatever I just wanted to hit it the old way and show them that I can hit the ball consistently when I swung the old way. But I had to practice perseverance so that the new way would pay off.

I knew from previous experience that I would feel the right way in my body eventually and I would then be able to let go of thinking. When you can hit by feeling the swing with your body then the consistency happens.

Sometimes we need to revisit stories of people who have achieved through great challenge and adversity. It helps boost our morale to not give up and not give in. When we are going through a hard time and adversity seems like the norm find encouragement in stories of others who had difficult encounters but achieved their dreams in the end. They can help keep you stay focused on a good attitude amidst disturbances around you. Helen Keller is one of my heroines for overcoming adversity and leaving behind a legacy of wisdom. I used to like reading the Chicken Soup for the Soul books here is one of her quotes I found in the second edition:

"The marvelous richness of human experience would lose something of the rewarding joy if there were no limitations to overcome. The hilltop hour would not be half so wonderful if there were no dark valleys to traverse."

– Helen Keller

There have been many times over the ten years, believe you/me that I wanted to chuck this concept and only teach yoga. I used to ask Spirit, "Why can't I just be a regular yoga teacher, why does it have to be for golfers?" The inner drive was always too strong to ignore. I would have to go back to teaching golfers to get any inner quiet. So my number one thing to do is ask the Goddess for support and it is always given. I may persistently ask the Goddess for a sign along the way and a coincidence will happen and I say great but there may still be fear about going in a certain direction. So I say, can you give me another sign, and I will get another and sometimes I still need more courage so I say "just one more" and you guessed another sign in the form of synchronicity comes. One reason I would ask for signs is because of all the resistance I would receive from family and friends. Some days it is hard to always be your own cheerleader so I would need the Goddess to help pump me up again. Another reason is I would be comparing myself and where I am in my journey. In the yoga world there is a saying "what we learn on the mat we take off the mat" Contentment instead of comparing is a big fundamental in yoga. It has probably been the hardest principle for me to integrate into my everyday life, since the act of comparing is so dominate in our society. I have always found the fable, *The Tortoise and the Hare* as a good reminder that the slow moving tortoise trusted that getting to the finish line did not have to be obtained quickly and immediately. He followed his own rhythm and pace. Nature's rhythms will work for us in the time and manner that is appropriate for us if we allow it. The lessons will be revealed in their own time as to why we had to move through the pressures of a particular moment. One of the pleasant discoveries I have found living in B.C. is that many tourists come here and so it is a wonderful chance to meet people from other countries. A woman I met recently, from England, said the same thing but in a different manner when we talked about what we each did for a living. She, like me, felt like she was going through a dark time. When we commented on why this happens she said, "How can you teach it if you don't go through it?" In her list of things she does, one of them is teaching meditation, but then she said, "Am I practicing it myself right now? No." I realize we humans can be lazy at times even when we have proof that yoga or any other holistic modality works it doesn't always mean we are on top of it.

When you do move away from it, then you can really see why you need it. For me, the poses have never been very important. I have not been interested teaching advanced Yoga, I like teaching beginner students. Generally golfers are perfect to teach because it is still a new discipline for them and they are not pushing for advanced yoga poses, but they are hungry for going into deeper teachings for the mind game. Now I see the importance of a disciplined practice for the body, since the death of my parents, traveling out west and more recently writing this book, my main discipline practice has been meditating and studying Raja Yoga. I have not practiced the poses in hatha yoga like I used to. I am living proof to myself that what you don't use you lose. My flexibility in my body is nowhere like it used to be. I have the experience of what it feels like to be in poses like twists and be relaxed. Now that I am back into my consistent hatha yoga practice I can easily preserve through the tight areas because I know the flexibility will come.

I have begun to feel the layers of tension in my shoulders beginning to give way and loosen up. With all the work on the computer I have accumulated much tightness in my neck and shoulders over the year and it feels good to begin to let it go. Because of not practicing my hatha yoga as much as my Raja yoga, there have been moments when I feel like a fraud. I have heard others comment on this in their own lives as well. We look like we are all together on the outside but we feel our life is falling apart on the inside. Most of us have to go through the dark night of the soul in our transformation of becoming. It is not a fun place but it is temporary, just like the high times of becoming, everything is temporary. We also may judge other yoga teachers we encounter, forgetting they are on the path as well, and some moments on the path are of struggle and pain. I remember one teacher promoting peace and hating her mother. I thought, "How could you be teaching about peace when you are at war in your family life?"

Now I realize that is exactly why she was teaching peace, the family was her catalyst to move her towards a higher vision. I have a better grasp on shifting to a higher awareness than when I first began yoga, I thought those who were on the path were filled with pure intentions and virtues. That is not always the case. Just because someone is saying they are on a spiritual path does not mean they are already healed. The interesting thing is that here in the West we are like infants when it comes to the spiritual path. In India the people know there are false prophets out there scamming people of their money, time and attention. There are people who may learn a trick or two of the yogic powers for their ego purposes so they look like they are evolved and powerful. The same can happen very easily over here. What I have done, and asked my students to do, is to go by Buddha's philosophy in which he said to his students after teaching them "Don't believe my words only, go out into the world and see if they are true for you".

Part 3
Direction West - Element Water

Goddesses of Water – Coventia a Scottish Goddess, Sedna an Inuit Goddess

- *Season: Fall*
- *Ceremony- Fall Equinox*
- *Quadrant of Day –Evening*
- *Stage of Life-Adulthood*
- *Color- Black*
- *Represents the Emotions*

Powers of the West- Adaptation, intuition, reflection, dreams, inner visions, emotions

Later adulthood the time of Fall, the time of the setting sun - twilight. The daylight fades and brings a new awareness in this time of gradual change. When the darkness comes we must look inward to find the light and have courage. To understand what we see in the darkness may not be real but only shadows. This is the emotional part of ourselves, like the flowing water we must learn to go with the flow of life. The time of the West is when we learn that we are responsible to all things and to each other. It is the time to prepare; to finish things for the time of winter is coming. We gather ourselves and family, working together to prepare for what is to come. As the place of emotions it is the place of family and love - of responsibility from our hearts because of the love. It is hard work and team efforts. Black symbolizes change from this life.

Yoga Poses for Water-pages **188-189**
Half Moon, Standing Yoga Mudra, Bridge, Frog, Spinal Twist

Chapter 5

Coventina– Scottish Water Goddess
Flexibility and Balance

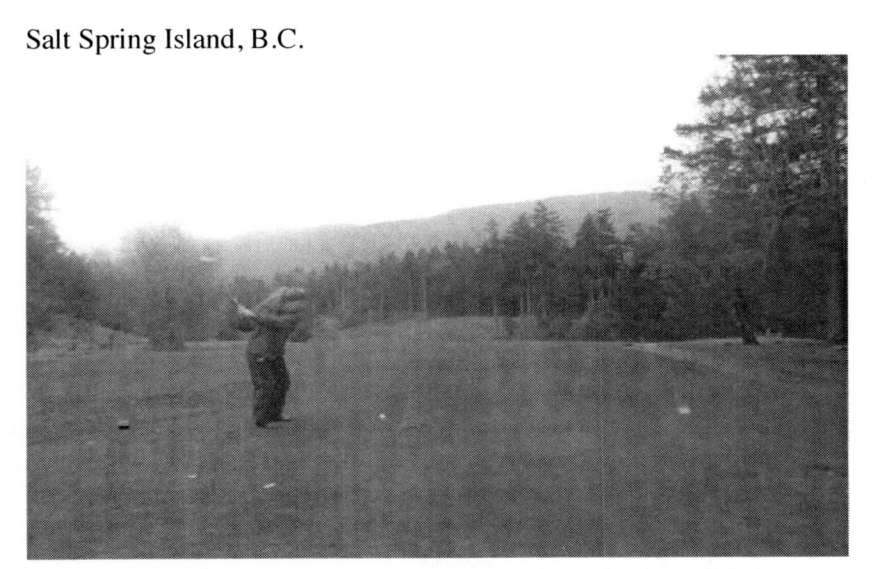

Salt Spring Island, B.C.

Me playing golf in the rain on the first day of winter/06

"Coventina is a goddess of rain, rivers, lakes, streams, ponds, oceans and water-based creatures. Because of her relationship to water, Coventina can swim into psychic domains and help with inspiration, psychic abilities, dreams and prophecies. She's also associated with purification and cleanliness, and you can call upon her for a spiritual baptism to relieve you of worries and judgments, and to help you abstain from unhealthful and addictive substances.

In ancient times, people would throw coins into a well associated with Coventina to request her assistance (this is believed to be the origin of the wishing well.). Because of the bounty of coins, Coventina represents abundance in all ways.

For today's modern women Coventina can be called on for abundance in closing a deal at the golf course.

Come, Be Golfing Goddesses!

Goddess Coventina representing the Front Nine

Hole 5 - Flexibility

"I am so happy to tell you that thanks to your classes, my handicap has gone from 20 to 16 and that I am enjoying golf again. Of course I still have bad rounds but can handle it much better now. I try and stay patient and "accept" instead of "expect."
  -Charlie Baker- Level 2 YFG.

    As we gain flexibility in our bodies we also gain it in our minds. With this flexibility we will find going with the flow of life and the direction of our games much easier to handle. Symbolically water has been associated with flow, fluidity and flexibility. In life, as well as on the golf course we aim for this flow, this flexibility; it is a power that others may classify as luck. Being flexible and able to adapt to change easily and effortlessly is essential for optimal performance and excellence in golf. A very beneficial habit to develop is to call to the Goddesses before playing golf to come help with your game. When you do this the shift is easily recognized in how much more smoothly the game goes. If you don't remember at first, you can call upon this energy to help whenever you start to become flustered or out of balance emotionally. You will find the effortlessness begin to happen whenever you call for guidance. This is a free-will universe we live in, there are many guides, angels, animal totems etc. that would love to help us humans, but we first need to make the request before they can.
    In the Native American tradition women are the keepers of water. It is women who offer the sacred tobacco to the water as a blessing. If you have read any of Masaru Emoto books on *'Messages in the Water'* he would agree with the Native American tradition. He tells us, 'that the whole human race will benefit by blessing the water." From a physical perspective human body is made up with a high percentage of water. Emoto experimented by placing words such as, 'you fool', or 'love', and 'gratitude' to the side of a container of water and then he would freeze the water. Using high- speed photography he would take a picture of the frozen

water and his book is filled with the pictures of formation of the crystals with positive words, music and images which all formed beautiful shapes.

Also with negative words, sounds and images that all made ugly and deformed shapes. This is the same thing that can happen inside our bodies since we are made up of mostly water, positive words are much healthier not only for our states of mind but now there is visual proof they effect our bodies as well.

Golfers do anything but bless the water on the golf courses. It is an obstacle, a challenge, a way to lose the game or a least gain extra scores that we don't want. This can be an ideal time to look at the lessons that come in the form of obstacles. Our society does not teach the value in making mistakes. But how do we gain experience and become wise? Through mistakes, obstacles, and suffering - we have a choice about how we go through hard times. These are character builders, just like golf can be if we play with awareness.

The hardest thing to do is to be grateful and bless our lessons when we are walking through them. If we begin on the golf course to bless the water each time we pass over it, not only are we beginning our own transformation but one with the earth as well. The lighter we walk upon the earth the more it heals. Each time we are faced with the challenge of getting our golf ball over the water, call upon Coventina for the courage to out-talk any negative chatter. Take a moment to capture in your imagination the shot you desire, visualize and feel the wonder of the shot. Then trust your body to deliver it.

Our connection with Coventina and other water Goddesses also ties into the connection with the Moon. You are my sisters; our cycles are linked to the Moon, and so are our moods. Like the changing Moon we have changing moods and bodies during a game, adaptation is a process of making specific adjustments in your attitude, approach and strategies when confronted by unpredictable changes before or during a game. The only true consistency I have found in golf is inconsistency. Events change quickly without warning.

Mother Nature has the power to change the weather at will regardless of what the weather predictions tell us. Maybe you have experienced this yourself while golfing? Golfers seem to be prepared to play in any kind of weather externally - they have golf umbrellas, waterproof shoes, rain gear packed in their golf bags along with sunscreen, and water. But many people are not prepared for change internally with the shifting weather patterns. Of course there are only fair weather golfers and if the weather man proves to be wrong and they get weather they were not expecting, than look out. Frustration, tension even anger can arise at the inconvenience. So which one are you? Can you generally stay calm and adapt to whatever golf gives you on a certain day, or are you in the later category. It helps to have this mantra, "It's not good or bad, it just is." Then use the mountain pose with the breath learned in chapter nine and you will gain an edge over someone who is resistant to unpredictable changes. Golf is all about challenge when you have challenge that means change. When you can adapt and accept any situation, you can stay relaxed and have a clear mental advantage over someone who is psychologically rigid or resistant.

In March 2003 I was teaching this flexibility of the mind theme when one of my students piped up and said they just had witnessed Tiger do the exact thing I was discussing, adapting. It was one of the weekend tournaments and on the last day of play he awoke with food poisoning. Tiger was going to go to the hospital instead of playing and his father said to him, " Remember Son, it is easy to get into the hospital, but it is hard to get out". So what did Tiger do - he adapted. He would hit the ball, then walk off the course to throw-up, hit the ball, throw-up. He did not become rigid, he stayed open and flexible AND ended up winning the tournament.

When we remain open and flexible it is easier to 'go with the flow' the exciting part is information comes our way effortlessly. Sometimes the tools we use don't seem like the right ones and someone will say something that you need exactly at that moment in time. It could just be a reminder of what you already know, but we are so close to our problems we can't see what is needed. We can get comfortable with our tools and by sharing other's viewpoints we gain a fresh perspective. The wonderful thing about sharing spiritual tools is that we never lose anything by doing it. We actually gain, as it makes us feel good to help others, and the lessons become deeper ingrained in ourselves.

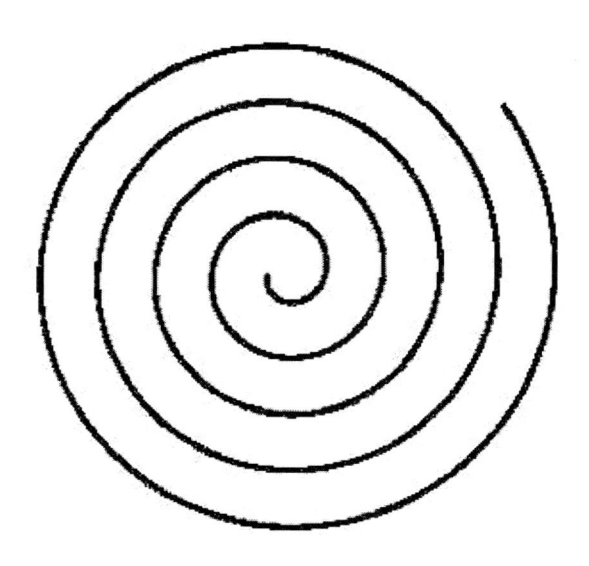

Goddess Coventina representing the Back Nine

Hole 14 - Balance

As the Goddess begins to rise again to help heal her children and this home we call Earth. I believe she will help us see our divinity as we connect back to her and learn from her in a whole new way. I believe we will all be living in a balanced way in equal partnership because we will have more of an understanding of energies that make up that Divine aspect of Goddess and God that we have right within us. Everything in nature has the feminine and masculine qualities moving within and without however humans are blessed with the ability to create our own worlds.

The symbol of yin and yang is balance, yin represents the feminine and the yang represents the masculine. Hatha Yoga translates to Ha meaning Sun and Tha meaning Moon. The meaning of Yin and Yang can also be symbolically viewed in the sun and moon, the right brain and left brain, and the East and the West. The feminine quality is the receptive one, the feeling, being, and channeling the Intuition from the Creatrix. It is associated with the East, Moon and the right brain. The masculine, the left logical brain, and the Sun all represent yang energy, this energy involves action, taking risks, movement; it is associated with the West. Someone out of balance who is using more masculine energy may be always doing but they may be spinning their wheels. They can't hear the voice of their spirit so many of the actions they do seem fruitless. If they would take time to be still they would get inspired to do the correct action and only have to do it once.

Someone who is more in touch with their feminine side may have all kinds of creative ideas but they do nothing about them, the ideas just sit on the shelf so to speak. Neither is very productive. When you are in balance you wait for the messages from the Universe by being still and receptive, a female trait, and then you engage the male side by take necessary actions and risks bring the message into physical form. The majority of times when we are practicing our preparation for the game it emulates the masculine, which is fine when first learning the game, but this endless physical practice of doing can be balanced with the female trait of being, using visualizations and creative right brain imagery.

For centuries our Goddess energy here in the West has been cut off or shut down. Not just in men but in women also. We have all been conditioned to be an intellectual society. On the inside cover of my golf C.D. I have put a well-documented soviet experiment.

Four matched groups of world class athletes were put on training programs prior to the 1980 Olympics. Group 1 trained only physically, group 2 trained physically 75% of the time and mentally 25% of the time. Group 3 divided physical and mental training equally, and group 4 put 25% into physical and 75% into mental. The athletes were evaluated and Group 1 doing only physical training showed the least improvement in performance. The group that showed the most improvement was the group that did the most mental training.

More and more Olympic athletes use the mental training of imagery and visualization. When I took my National Coaching program they showed us a movie on how skaters will first visualize themselves doing a jump in their minds first, then they would execute it physically. It was a two step process that they would repeat over and over. So my question then to you is, "Have you been playing golf like a man? Do you only practice physically?" Another imbalance in the way most men view golf courses they are out to conquer it instead of yielding to it. Do you have this mind set as well?

With a new perception gained from this book you will be able to release that mindset. If we approach the golf course as our Mother Earth that we are playing upon and we are showing up to learn from her it is easier to yield right from the get go. As mentioned under setting goals and the relaxation chapter it is by surrendering to the game and the earth that brings the Power not by force or domination. Some of the Goddesses in this book have a warrior quality but that is used to conquer the inner bad habits, not to be a warrior over others or nature. In this chapter we use the essence of water to be fluid like a willow tree in the wind, which bends and sways with the wind, not like a solid oak whose branches can snap off. We have been disconnected with nature for so long we don't even know how to learn from her anymore. What are the lessons we need to be watching for? One is simplicity, we have become so out of balance with our cultural materialism that this is carried over into the sports we play or the pastimes we are meant to enjoy. We don't need many of the gadgets that can burden us down for a day of being in Nature. The most important and powerful tools to feel better and play better are within each of you. I'm not suggesting that you have to give up anything all at once.

When you find out for yourself that most of the advertised gadgets are just money- making schemes you will let them drop naturally from your life. Think of the term 'less is more' and you will find more balance and harmony with your game, especially when it comes to using less of the logical, analytical mind and using your more of your creative, mystical, magical mind.

Today I am using the golf course to over-emphasize living in the wonder by playing the game. I think of myself as a child again and it makes me feel lighter as I am coming more from an open heart. It would be easier if my playing partners had the same mindset but it doesn't matter. When I think of children playing, the most dominant quality is their curiosity; they like to imagine all kinds of stories. While playing golf the other day I told myself on the drive to the course that it was going to be a beautiful, magical day. Then I looked for signs to confirm this, when I accentuate the positive and eliminate the negative I can live more in my heart. On one of the holes my ball landed near a creek and as I walked up to it I saw some twigs and grasses stuck between some rocks and there were little sparkles of light.

Now my magical thinking said, "Oh the fairies are here", and I said hello to them and went on to hit my ball. I could have just as easily thought from my left-brain and said, "Oh there are water droplets caught in the grass and the position I am standing in shows the sun's prism through the droplets." But what fun would that be. We have a choice on how we want to view anything in life. And since we are conditioned to think with the analytical mind, it takes practice to live in the heart. We may have to over-emphasize our imagination at first until we come to a balance between the mind and the heart. There is a great line in one of Van Morrison's songs I would like to share with you;

> *"If my heart could do my thinking*
> *and my head began to feel,*
> *I could look upon the world and you*
> *and see what's truly real."* -Van Morrison

What is true is that there is a new Earth being birthed, the old paradigms are falling away. A great prophecy of balance comes from South America called "The Eagle and the Condor." I found one description on-line with permission to use it in its entire content. You will understand more if you Google- "The Eagle and The Condor" -

"We have been waiting five hundred years.
The Inca prophecies say that now, in this age, when the eagle of the North and the condor of the South fly together, the Earth will awaken. The eagles of the North cannot be free without the condors of the South.
Now it's happening. Now is the time. The Aquarian Age is an era of light, an age of awakening, an age of returning to natural ways. Our generation is here to help begin this age, to prepare through different schools to understand the message of the heart, intuition, and nature. Native people speak with the Earth. When consciousness awakens, we can fly high like the eagle, or like the condor...

Ultimately, you know, we are all native, because the word native comes from nature, and we are all parts of Mother Nature. She is inside us, and we are inside her. We depend totally on the Earth, the Sun, and the Water. We belong to the evolution of nature in our physical bodies. But we also have a spiritual body that comes from the Sun, not the Sun you can see with two eyes, but another Sun that lies in another dimension, a golden Sun burning with the fire of spiritual light. The inner light of humans emanates from this spiritual source. We came to Earth from this Sun to have experiences on Earth, and eventually we will return to this Sun. We are Children of the Sun."
  - Willaru Huayta is an Incan Spiritual Messenger from Cusco, Peru. Born a Quechua Indian, he learned to receive esoteric truth during his spiritual quests in the Amazon jungles.

Part of taking time off from the rat race and living in trust that my partner and I will be provided for I have followed the lessons in Nature. Life has turned through the seasons and kept me involved while giving me the space while I wrote. Sometimes in our lives we are in total balance with the seasons sometimes it seems we need to live the major lessons by living in the energies of one season for a longer stretch of time. It seems most of our society is comfortable living in the energies of the Spring and Summer season, the action or Yang energy. The part I have been living in for the past few years is the lessons from the Winter season, which is going within and living the Hermit life. The winter teaches us to be still and allow your path to reveal itself to you. It is known as old man winter but I think it is grandmother because when we are still and receptive we are living in the feminine quality.

This applies to whether we are men or women because it is the energy that is within all things. There is a cycle or time of doing and one of being, one thing I have noticed is that many New Years resolutions fail because they are actually going against the natural rhythm and this leaves many people feeling bad or shameful. This habit can be broken with understanding. The reason people fail is because it is still the winter energy and their bodies still need to be in rest mode. Never mind that most people's bodies, mind and emotions are recovering from the hectic month of December. The Spring Equinox is a more suitable time to be making goals not because it is the season of the East and it represents new beginnings but through my own experience I have noticed the energy in my body awakening, it is so much easier to begin new projects because there is more power and energy within the mind and body to get up and go so goals do not fall by the wayside like they do in January.

Chapter 6

Sedna – Inuit Water Goddess
Intuition and Focus

Poem to Sedna
My fingers were cut off then I was kicked
I was hurt
I was wounded
I was lied to
I was betrayed
I was abandoned
My suffering was great
but down below in the deeps
in the heart of the ocean
where I was left to die
I realized my powerlessness
the way my life was lived
helpless and afraid
always being done to
instead of doing
and saw what I did
As realization expanded my consciousness
fish and sea mammals
grew out of my cut fingers
I became "old food dish"
She who provided for her people
Victim no more

Myth - The Inuit of North America called their sea Goddess Sedna (pronounced sed'nah). Sedna was once a beautiful woman who was not satisfied with the many suitors who courted her. Wooed by a seagull with promises of plenty of food and servants, she went to live with the bird people. Instead of the promised conditions, she was forced to live in filth and squalor. When her father came for a visit, she begged him to take her back home with him across the waters.

The bird people pursued them and to save his life, her father threw Sedna overboard. When she tried to climb back into the boat, he cut off her fingers. Sedna's cut fingers transformed into fish and sea mammals.

The Lessons of this Goddess

Sedna swims into your life to tell you to stop being a victim. The way to wholeness is to recognize how you've been caught up in and are living the victim archetype, then to change the pattern by empowering yourself. Are you fond of saying, "Why is this happening to me?" Don't get stuck in the "why". Look realistically at what you are creating, than you can work to change it. Do you feel your needs are too insignificant to negotiate? Does everyone in your life seen to take advantage of you? Your way to wholeness lies in recognizing when you are playing the victim and stopping it. Sedna says we have all been victimized by something, by patriarchal institutions, discrimination based on race, gender, sexual preference, religion, or color. She encourages you to claim your power. The Goddess says you are too precious and necessary in this dance of life to waste valuable energy and time being a victim. Rather than dissipating your energy, create what you want.

http://www.angelfire.com/va/goddesses/sedn.html

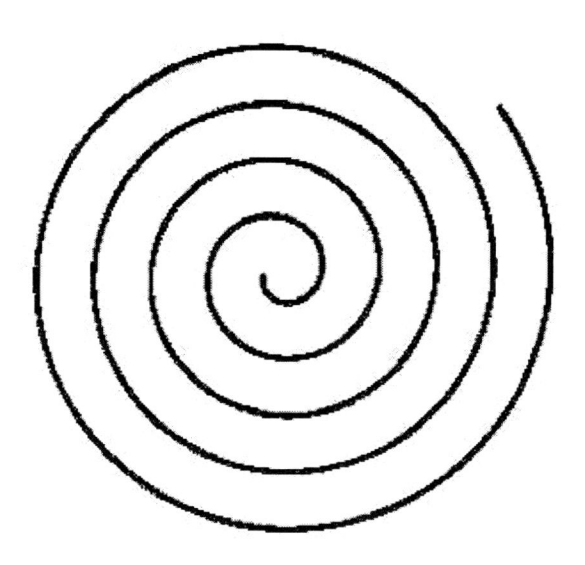

Goddess Sedna representing the Front Nine

Hole 6 - Intuition

To begin the road to self-love and to leave the victim road behind it is helpful to fully embrace your womanhood. As a child I always wanted to be a boy. I have three brothers and no sisters and I felt left out of doing many fun things because I was a girl.

My parents passed the message on to me that because I was a girl I was not good enough. I don't think they did it intentionally but that is what I grew up believing. Now I am so happy I am not a male in this changing world. How do we claim our power and love ourselves? I am going to share something from my sacred bundle on polar bear because this chapter is using the teachings of an Inuit Goddess and bear is in the direction of the west.

In the Native Path each direction has an animal associated with it. I have heard Polar Bear called into the direction of the North by some people. I have since learned that different tribes have different animals for each direction so the only consistency is inconsistency.

I'm sad to say I've had this message on bear for this so long I don't know who wrote it or where I got it from however the words are very empowering I had to add it to the book.

"To express yourself in strength, conviction and with no apologies for being who you are, you radiate the confidence of Bear. Our energy is fearless, powerful, confident and graceful. Our appearance may belie the grace and speed of our actions, but our inner confidence and pose allows us to be all things.

Express yourself without apology. Be willing to make mistakes and learn from them.

You are who you are. And that is good enough. We are Bear. Live our confidence, grace and power and you take on Bear energy. Be like us."

When we begin to come out of the darkness and fully into the light it is hard to stay there. Many times I hear women say, "Things are going so well, I'm sure my luck will change any day now." I would give many of my classes another hand-out I acquired somewhere along the way. It has always moved my student's, see if it does the same for you?

Light
Our deepest fear is not that we are inadequate.
Our deepest fear is that we are powerful beyond measure.
It is our light, not our darkness that frightens us.
We ask ourselves,
Who am I to be brilliant, gorgeous, talented, and fabulous?
Who are you not to be?
You are a child of God.
Your playing small does not serve the world.
There is nothing enlightened about shrinking so that other people won't feel insecure around you.
We were born to make manifest the glory of God within us. It's not just in some of us, it's in everyone. And as we let our own light shine, we unconsciously give other people permission to do the same. As we are liberated from our own fear, our presence automatically liberates others.
-Nelson Mandela, 1994 Inaugural Speech

Living in the light develops naturally as we follow our inner promptings, our common sense, our instincts and intuitive intelligence. I am going to tell you the difference between intuition and instinct from my own personal experience. It is close to what I have read and researched over the years and I'm not sure which came first, the reading on how to follow my intuition or the confirmation that I was on the right path by the books I was reading. A funny thing that happens to me is I have always been a magnet to the right books at the right time. For me Intuition can be a direction from our future selves.

For example at the time I was writing this chapter we were deciding to move once again from the wonderful Island of Salt Spring, B.C. to more of the city life in North Vancouver, so I ask for confirmation from the universe in the form of signs or symbols so I know I am following the right path. The owl is one of my totems and has shown itself over and over again on what path to take. I even have a picture of me taken with an owl when I went to the Golf Show in Vancouver, just after asking the question (for the umpteenth time) "Am I really to move away from Salt Spring?" and the Outdoor show was being held at the same time in another part of the building.

Come, Be Golfing Goddesses!

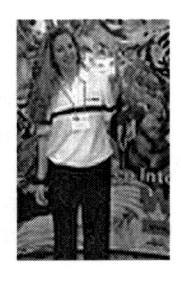

I went to the bathroom and when I came back I was putting my purse below my table and when I stood up, a woman was at my booth with a falcon on her wrist. I was a bit startled and then she just pips up that I can get my picture taken with an owl if I go to the Vancouver Zoo booth on the other side. Wow, that was clear. I have now moved, but it was something in the future for me at the time so my intuition was guiding me forward into my future.

On the golf course or while living moment to moment my instincts come more into play. My goal is to get more holes-in-one so I may come to a par three, and I read the yardage and I think I know what club to use and my gut feeling will prompt me to use another. If I doubt, I lose out. I have been giving my sub-conscious the vision and if I don't listen to the prompting I am in essence saying I don't trust myself. The more I listen to my inner promptings the stronger and more intense the messages become.

The first thought is usually the highest thought, the one from spirit. The second and third are the doubts of the logical, lower mind. Some people believe they can only ask for help of advice for important issues not for areas like playing. What you must remember is what ever you desire starts from inside of you so you are always in a partnership and the sacred exists all day long in everything and everyway. The more we can practice listening and trusting the little things the easier it will be for the bigger things in life.

Your body is your best friend, it has a built in protection system, a radar. Even if you don't listen to it, it always will always stand by you and forever help and love you.

"All the women leaders I have met led with a greater sense of intuition than men. I am almost completely intuitive. The only time I've made a bad business decision is when I didn't follow my instinct. My favorite phrase is: "Let me pray on it." Sometimes I literally do pray, but sometimes I just wait to see if I wake up and feel the same way in the morning. For me, doubt normally means don't. Doubt means do nothing until you know what to do. And I'm really, really, really attuned to that."

-Oprah Winfrey on Leading Women:
How I Got There - online Newsweek

I have found it interesting the different ways I have connected with my sisters while doing the Goddess Yoga classes compared to the Yoga for Golf. As a group, not only do we bond more but it is as if our intuition builds and expands as a group.

It is similar to when a group of women are living together and their moon time comes at the same time each month.

    I must take time to mention a very special woman who has been tuned into me over the years. Her name is Diane Pitcher and she took my Yoga for Golf class at her golf club in Oakville, Ontario, back in 1998. I have told her over and over again that she contacts me right when I need a boost to keep teaching Yoga for Golf. Many times over the years I have wanted to give up as there seemed to be no progress in golfers embracing this program. I have moved a couple of times and she has always found me. It is easier now that I have a website with my email address but still, even moving out to B.C. I have received emails from her staying in touch. I call her my earth angel because of the uncanny intuition she has to call or email me exactly when I need encouragement to keep going.

    I decided that I would ask her some questions since I am writing my book. On July 2, 2007 I emailed her these questions and added her replies.

> *Margarit-* When did you start doing yoga?
>
> *Diane-* I started doing yoga in the mid 80's
>
> *M-*Did you find a difference between general yoga and Yoga for Golf?
>
> *D-*Yes, I did find a difference. Regular yoga concentrates on postures and breathing – more physical, whereas YFG concentrates on physical but more on the MENTAL aspect.
>
> *M-*when did you first take up golf, and how old are you now?
>
> *D-*I was in my late 40's and I am now ,,74
>
> M-do you still remember the tools of YFG and do you still use them to day?
>
> *D-* Yes, I still remember the tools- especially the centering (the circle with the thumb and finger). The RELAX as you swing through the ball. A good deep breath in and out before you swing. Affirma tions- believing that I am A GREAT GOLFER!!!! And I am!!
>
> *M-* You have a telepathic link to me. When I am about to give up YFG you always contact me, can you explain it?
>
> *D-* I don't really know how to explain it- but somehow there is a con nec tion. Without realizing it I probably contact you or try to find you when things are not the best for me. You are very calming. Make any sense?

It is very confirming to me and should be for you that these are easy steps I am teaching here and as Diane mentions she is still using them nine years later. Many times our intuition doesn't seem to make sense to ourselves or to others at the time but every action, whether we are aware of it or not, sends a ripple out into the universe.

The element of water is associated with the emotions in the human body. Emotions in relation to yoga are part of the healing process. I have taught many classes where beginning students cry when we do the final relaxation. I myself have gone into a pose and burst out crying for no reason that I know of. My teachings tell me that all memory is stored in our cells and sometimes we can go into a movement that releases a painful memory from the body, although the mind might not recall or doesn't judge it to be important enough to cry about. I was never taught that crying was good as a child.

Through conditioning I see how out of balance I was growing up, because I would never cry. I have since learned that tears are very healing and I now allow them to wash through me when they come up. I now believe in this quote from a Chinese proverb, "Tears are to the soul what soap is for the body." I recognize that at certain times of the month I am more weepy or tired and that has to do with my menstrual flow. Now that I have more understanding of our connection as women to the moon, emotions, water and our menstrual cycles I take more responsibility for myself. I had read for many years that a good practice to get to know myself would be to I chart my monthly flows on my calendar, which I have begun to practice, and it is very helpful. When I see my time approaching I will take more B vitamins for the bitchiness or rest so I am more in balance and taking care of my body. Just by doing this one simple act keeps the household more in harmony. I have found that in the house it is me that sets the tone for the rest of the family. When I have more balance and peace so does everyone else.

I am being prompted to add one more piece that happen in Aug. 2008 when Native Elder Dave Courchene came to do ceremonies in North Vancouver (a full introduction of him is under Earth and Gaia). I had asked if he would do a water Ceremony and he graciously agreed. At the water ceremony Dave spoke about many important aspects of water he related how women are close to this element and it is water that surrounds babies and is the first thing to come before the baby. Dave then felt it necessary to tell all of us gathered that he feels the biggest mistake his people have made has been not to listen to women, the mothers and grandmothers. He then included this same mistake for all men. He encouraged all of us women to begin to step up. He told us he sees this time and the coming future as the time for women to lead from the gifts our own true being." As nurturers, as the connectors we naturally are since women are closely connected to the Earth.

He used his pipe to bless the water and while he was doing so he asked us to bless the containers of water we each brought. He asked us to add our heartfelt feelings of love and gratitude for water, this simple act I have since been repeating whenever I am by water and I have a water bottle. I add love and gratitude and then pour some into the water. I have been in many ceremonies but I have never felt the oneness and Love flowing through a group like it did this day, it is exciting to experience the oneness and break through the illusion that we are all separate. Then he had the women and girls lead down to the water and empty our containers first, and the men to follow. Dave and others who are channels for the earth want us to know, all humans are loved so much by nature. Everything in the natural world desires to be back in connection with us, back in harmony. Each time we pay attention to nature, nature pays attention back to us in very recognizable ways that they we are heard. The healings we do for this planet do make a difference. The twenty or so of us that gathered and blessed the water did make a difference and I was shown the sign the very same day; It was an overcast day with periods of rain but around dinner the sun came out to reveal a rainbow, the sign for hope. It made me think about what Dave said at least three times to the group,"

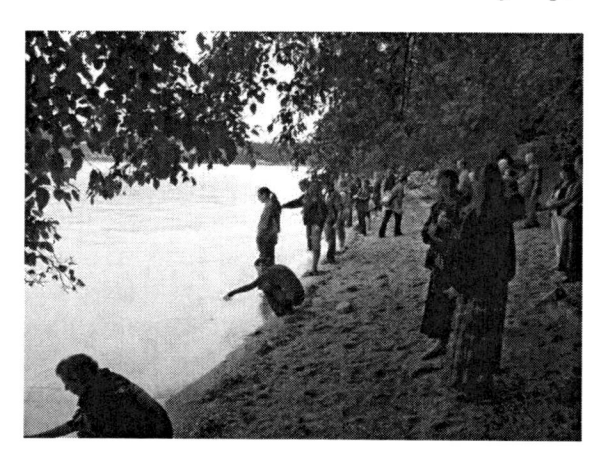

"Do not under estimate the power of our work today." He asked us to "THINK BIG". To understand that the ripple effects going into the ocean today will spread out to other waters, the blessings will go into the clouds and then when it rains the blessings will shower down on everything.

I have seen we are all capable of many great things. It is not science and technology that is going to help us soar to the skies, or the images of space shows that beckon us to use technology to transport people. NO, it is our own spiritual nature that is right within our beings, we can learn to do many things (like flying) by becoming connected to our source. We still have not tapped into our richness, our full capabilities, we just keep creating things outside of ourselves that we as humans are capable of doing right within.

Think about computers and how we are connected by the internet. I wrote on my sacred connections blog for the 2008 fall equinox that a Goddess who is evidently influencing our lives right now is Grandmother Spider, the web is connecting us to the world. Spider was said to have given humans the first alphabet through the designs in their webs. We are using the written word as the dominate way to communicate with the World. If you are educated about the new children, the Indigos, you will know that they come into this world with the ability to communicate internally, they are all connected to a web that they use to communicate with one another, they do not need technology. Everyone has this same capability, as adults we have to work to uncover it and through practice it will grow stronger, just like a muscles in the body the same applies to our energy and sixth sense. However, I have noticed in the 14 years since my Yoga Teacher Training that as more people work on themselves the shifts have become faster and shorter. What affects one person affects everyone.

Are you ready to THINK BIG?

When one is living close to the Earth, the earth will reveal what a person or people need. When our ancestors had dreams of what plants to eat and what to avoid it was Nature that took care of them. Not through synthetic drugs but plants and herbs. There is a plant from the Amazon that is calling out to people of this modern day. And people from all over this planet are traveling to South America to work with the plant and the Shamans. This is a fast forward experience into the heart and out of the head, to help people move through this difficult era and break away from former conditioning.

This plant is Ayahuasca, it is very ancient and very wise, you would be amazed at how much one plant can impart wisdom, healing and awakening. The risk and trusting for my partner and I to embark on the journey to Brazil and work with the Shaman was the scariest thing we had ever done and also the most magical. Although it is too much detail for this book, if you find it interesting and want more information www.heartoftheintitiate.com are the people who arranged it all and even have recorded teachings from the Shaman on the website. This again is exciting evidence that the prophecy of "The Eagle and the Condor" it is happening now, the Eagle people who are developed with technology can now bring forth the teachings of the Condor, the people who have developed Spiritually together for the benefit of everyone. Please recognize that directions are not relative per say there are many Condor's living in all across the globe and many in North America.

Goddess Sedna representing the Back Nine

Hole 15 - Focus

A simple method to develop focus and concentration naturally occurs by balancing the body via yoga poses such as the Tree Pose. Learning to focus on the golf course can begin at the driving range and using the markers as targets. That is why they are there; mini putt also has examples of having to stay focused by the swinging bar across the hole and other obstacles. Do you have fun doing this? We want to aim at the target every time in golf what is the target, the flag! If you can't see the flag then aim at some distant spot to first get you close to the pin, in other words do not even acknowledge any hazards such as the water or the bunker. The golf channel once said that Ben Hogan admitted "if he had his career to do over again, he would aim at the pin every time." To become a pin seeker takes focus and discipline.

You have probably learned by now that yoga is a discipline, it is 5,000 years old. The D word did not mean drudgery it was a matter of living a better life. The caste system of India kept people in one lifestyle their entire lives. The yogis were forest dwellers who left the caste system to prove that anyone can reach fulfillment and enlightenment, one did not have to wait until reincarnation to become the highest caste the Brahmin (priests). Yoga has scientific results if you do one thing you will get a certain result. These results have been tested twice over first in India and now in here west. I recently found out that the word science actually means that which works. I know that yoga is not a passing fad because it works anyone who has ever given it a proper chance knows it works. There is nothing to prove it is a science.

However, if you do find it hard to believe that a culture behind our times in technology are worthy of scientific proof then I suggest reading the book *"Autobiography of a Yogi"* by Parahamansa Yoganada. This book has wonderful examples of not only great Indian Scientists but of Yogis disciplining their minds to create what we the average person would consider miracles. Although the book 'A Course in Miracles' explains the meaning of a miracle is, *"miracles are a change of perception'*. We have a modern day yogi in the discipline of Raja Yoga named Chris Angel he calls himself 'The Mind Freak' you may have heard of him, and his show. If he can do these things we all can but who wants to work that hard on mental training? We don't have to discipline as much as he does, but to live happier, freer lives we must gain control and let go at the same time. The process begins with a desire and willingness to go through the personal growth with focus and training, clearing out the old to make way for the new.

Today you only have to read any of Jon Kabbit–Zins books to have documented proof of the power of the mind to heal and this is used in hospitals very successfully. If you can aim at your target and stay focused you can then use the discipline to turn fear into excitement. Let's say one of your goals is to be on the LPGA tour. By the time you are ready to go on tour and have a crowd watching you will have believed in yourself enough to know you belong on the tour.

You can't think of failure or mistakes, set backs will happen but that just means there is more to learn it does not mean failure. Pro Golfer Kathy Whitworth said, *"Golf is a game of misses and the winners are those who have the best misses."* A great exercise to help you focus is to use a visualization that you are on tour. See yourself matched up in a tournament with your favorite pro, visualize or feel yourself playing beautifully. Vision boards are popular these days that is because they work! Having a vision board of everything you would experience as a touring pro helps it not only come to pass one day but you will know you can handle it. How? It will not seem so unfamiliar to you if you are in the pictures and you look at the board frequently. The attitude to have here is one of gratitude.

At all times you want to be having fun. This is a game you are playing, and the preparation can become a game as well. Training you to stay focused on complete awareness of each present moment as it is unfolding. By being grateful of the beauty in nature know that you are full of greatness as you are a part of nature, when you stay focused on this aspect the golf course will revel to you, your greatness.

I read on a greeting card - *"there are only two things worth striving for in life, the first is to get what you want and the other is to enjoy it when you get it."* When you are focused you remember that you are here to enjoy what you have. In the game it is to focus fully on the present moment each time you play and are in nature.

I will share a story how of two dogs displayed the lesson of focus for me and by watching them I once again noticed the proper steps involved in attaining a goal. I watched them playing at ocean shore with their owner and the cool part was this occurred while I was writing about this theme on focus. I was also reading a book that encouraged people to stay focused and true to their dreams, and to not let failure or defeat become a distraction, because so many people have given up or quit their goals or dreams just before success came.

Come, Be Golfing Goddesses!

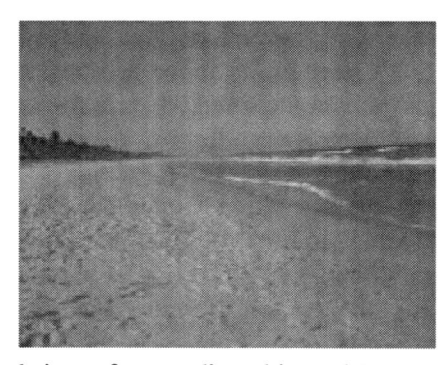

I was at the beach just after reading this and I watched how these two dogs were intently focused when sticks were being thrown in the water. There were many other dogs at the beach and they never got distracted by any of them as they came over to play. One dog was older and definitely more focused and persistent. At one point he lost sight of a stick that was thrown out too far and then the stick floated farther away with the current. This dog swam and swam looking for the stick. He started swimming up and away from the flow of the current as his stick floated farther away in the opposite direction. His owner first tried to get him going in the right direction then started to cal him back to shore. But the dog would have nothing to do with the orders became obvious that he would not return to shore until he had a stick to bring back with him.

It was amazing to watch his energy to keep going, and it was funny to see him keep swimming in the wrong direction. But then he found another stick floating by and he brought that back to his owner. The lesson he portrayed was he did bring a stick back which was his goal, even if it wasn't the original one and he got it by going the wrong way. So how do we stay focused when we can't see the road and it seems like we are stuck and going nowhere or going the wrong way? A simple but effective way is to begin to heighten our awareness so we can hear our true nature which always guides even if it looks like we going the wrong way to our logical minds.

Meditation, creative visualization and affirmations are ways to heighten our awareness. I was listening to a yoga teacher give a talk about the benefits of meditation. He said when we meditate our path gets lit up, we begin to change the channel in our heads to tune into higher vibrations and then the still small voice becomes louder. This way we begin to trust and follow the messages even if they look ridiculous to our logical minds. He went on to describe our trusting in the metaphor of driving your car on the freeway. You are listening to the news and they say that the road you are on is piled up with cars because of an accident and to take an alternate route. So what do you do? The road is clear where you are but up ahead it is stopped.

Now you can't see that it is stopped but you trust the voice on the radio and you take the next cut off to avoid being stopped in traffic. This act is trusting what is not before our eyes the same way that it can happen when you are focusing your mind on your higher truer states of being.

This same methodology of trusting can be transferred into our golf games by not judging what the eyes are showing us at any given time throughout our game. Because the game is always changing and if we have stayed focused throughout the year with a goal, say to have more eagles in our rounds, then the eagles can come on any given hole, the trick is staying relaxed and focusing only on one shot at a time. It is helpful to train the mind first to focus and concentrate before jumping into meditation. A very effective concentration exercise is candle gazing.

Heightening Intuition through candle gazing.

1. Place a lighted candle in front of you. Approx 2 feet. Gaze directly at the flame for a few minutes working up to two.
2. Begin by pressing palms up to closed eyes to see the image of the flame. The flame may bounce around from left to right. But bring it to the middle as much as you can. The point between your eyebrows.
3. With practice you will be able to see it clearly without putting your palms on your eyes.
4. Begin to count how long you can hold the image of the flame or the col or's it changes to. Each time you practice it will stay longer and longer.

A guru would tell you that humans have two minds a higher and a lower and the more we can raise our gaze to the point between the eyebrows the more we naturally develop our higher mind and live from the higher states.

There are many methods by which we can pacify and tame the lower mind and activate and awaken the higher mind. One of the best ways to do this is to focus the attention at the eyebrow center, also called the third eye. This is the point that controls all the levels of the mind, both lower and higher. When it is stimulated by yogic and meditative processes, it calms the thoughts and emotions and allows the deeper and subtler intuitive elements to manifest.

Part 4
Direction North - Element Earth

Goddesses of Earth –
Gaia and Artemis both Greek Goddesses

- Season: Winter
- Ceremony- Winter Solstice
- Quadrant of Day –Night
- Stage of Life-Elderhood
- Color- White
- Represents the Body

Powers of the North- Grounding, roots, growth, blooming and manifestation

Earth element is symbolic of wisdom, patience, manifesting and prosperity.

As we get older our hair turn white, as we come to our time of winter. White (and purple) also symbolizes spirituality. With experience and age we gain wisdom. Now we have time to rest and contemplate the lessons. North is purity and wisdom, a great place of healing. This is the time after midnight, a dream time. The time to be grounded within yourself and deep within, like a bear in a cave. North is the place of winter. This reminds us to stop and listen. That we must have prepared for the long time of winter. Having been in action the other seasons we now rest and contemplate to understand the wisdom we have been given.

Yoga Poses for Earth- pages **190-194**
Tree, Chair, Dancer, Forward Bends - Turkish Grounding- pages 153 -159

Chapter 7

Gaia – Greek Earth Goddess Mother Earth and Sacred Play

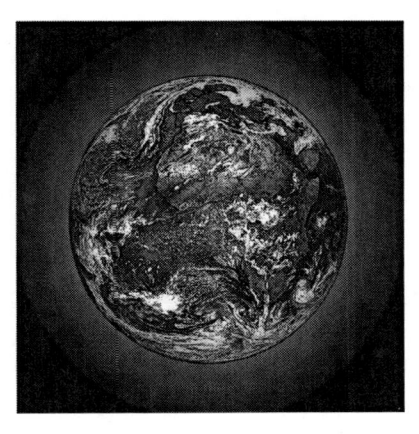

Gaia is a Greek goddess known as earth or mother earth.
The Greek common noun for "land" is GE or GA

Gaia Symbols - Earth, Grounding, Foundation, Our Bodies, Connection to golf - Beauty of the golf courses, the different grass and shapes of the fairways and greens. Feel the Earth beneath our feet, feel the earth when replacing divots

The Sacred Earth

"The goddess is the earth itself, the personification of Nature.
She gives birth to all her children, feeds and nourishes them
And takes them back to her body when they die.
Through the generosity of the earth mother the land is fertile and food
is Plentiful."

Come, Be Golfing Goddesses!

Goddess Gaia representing the Front Nine

Hole 7 - Mother Earth

Gaia- "She is the gentle caretaker of planet earth. Scientists have proven that the earth is a living, pulsating breathing organism.

Earth as a living entity, earth has its own rhythm and its own divine magic within it.

We all have the ability to communicate with non-human entities and the earth is the oldest and the wisest. This ability already exists for each of us. Especially as women, we are closer to the earth and it only needs be discovered and used. When you play golf you are playing the game upon the Mother Earth and it is important to connect back to the land and learn from her as much as we can. The lessons from the earth can give us directions to playing the game of life. Let's think of the golf courses as feminine, because they are, they are the Earth. This is a magical planet we live upon and we can experience magical golf games if we approach the golf course with an open heart to learn from Gaia.

> "If you pay no attention to the cycles and seasons of life and the energies they call into play, you will be constantly surprised, and not always happily, with what "Lady Luck" brings you."
> - Carol Bridges

We in the west are conditioned to go after the direct line to the next step to success. However, this is not the lesson we learn from our Mother. And as my own mother always said to me: "Life is one-step forward two steps backward." When we start believing in the signs from spirit it gives us courage to face the backward steps. As we ground our intention that we are playing upon our home, our ultimate mother, golf games can take on a more respectful and loving approach making our golf sacred play.

I am happy to mention that golfers are raising the awareness throughout the world today for preserving the land and our home. One company, Audubon International, is supporting golf courses to be eco-friendly. There are now 50 golf courses in Canada that are eco-friendly supporting a natural environment for waterfowl by cutting back on watering and the use of pesticides and herbicides. To learn more go to about becoming a green golfer go to www.audoboninternational.org.

> *"I am only one, but still I am one,*
> *I cannot do everything, but still I can do something,*
> *I will not refuse to do the something, I can do."*
> Helen Keller

When you begin to feel a connection with the earth and all the kingdoms within it, you will recognize you are never alone. This planet, our ultimate home, is really a friendly place. We've just lost touch with this truth or perhaps we were never taught to think this way. We only have to look to the animals to see that the earth does provide for them with everything they need. The same is true for us and we only have to wake up to this fact that everything we have and even our bodies our made from the earth and her elements.

Since I moved to British Columbia and taken time out to write, I have been more in tune with nature. One little bird that sings, I believe it is a finch. It keeps teaching me to be *right here*. Its song is one of chirping a bit and then it ends with a long two whistles that sound like the words "Right Here". This is such a great message, the few little chirps is a reminder to me that my head can go off chattering and then I must bring it back to Right Here. A common message from many spiritual teachings is to be in the now, the present moment.

That is always your point of power since the past and the future are out of our control and it is hard to enjoy being in nature if our head is bent on thoughts like, doing chores, the shopping, paying bills, or any number of things we can choose to worry about throughout the day. Give yourself permission for a time-out when you are out in nature. Look, listen and learn from Nature - she has many secrets to reveal.

I have always loved being in nature and I was reintroduced to the magical connection of Mother Earth from a Native Elder many years ago. I resonated immediately with his teachings that centered around having a great love and respect for Gaia and also for women and children. I was first introduced to this Elder and the Native Ceremonies in 1995 while I was also taking my Yoga Teacher Training. I just had a physic reading a few months before meeting him and I was told that I was a native in my past life and it would help me quicker along my path in this life time if I was to study the Native Traditions. Now I was open to this because I was learning about reincarnation through the yoga path. Someone in my yoga class brought in a flyer about a three-day weekend to learn from a Native Man who would lead us in the sweat lodge and sunrise ceremony. I did not know the people running the event and it was a good two hours from my home. The woman who brought in the flyer could not go and I was scared to go by myself, but my intuition kept pushing me to go.

I gathered up all my courage and went away for the weekend, all on my own. This was a big step for me back then, leaving my former husband at home with the kids and not even taking a friend with me. I came away from that weekend realizing I had just taken the first big step in trusting my intuition and it became the beginning of living a better life for me. I discovered a whole new way of perceiving life around me. Most of what I experienced could not be explained intellectually it was more of a feeling of coming home.

To introduce his teachings to this book I draw upon my journal. I had begun journaling daily a couple of years before I had met him, so I had bought a new journal that was especially for this introduction into the Native path, which has become my ceremonial journal. The writing of this book has helped reveal a gift to me that was always there but I did not fully recognize until now. That I am a recorder, a record keeper or I would have been called a story teller in Native tradition.

You see when Dave gave his teachings it was around the sacred fire, one does not write while in ceremony it is a time for being, listen, learning. As another elder taught me, "learn to listen, listen to learn." We went to the fire each morning and evening for teachings and then I would go back to my tent and write down what Dave had said. Whenever I have revisited this journal I always see the truth of his words and now recognize him as a visionary. Over the years I have had an opportunity to be in ceremony with this wonderful holy man many times and each time is more powerful then the last. He is from Manitoba but he made the trips to Ontario many times and in 2008 came to B.C.

As a full introduction to this man I give you his Christen name and his native name: Dave Courchene Jr. his native name is, Nii Gaani Aki Inini, in English it translates to 'Leading Earth Man' he is a leader who is descended from a long line of leaders and chiefs of his people. Dave learned the significance of the fire through a personal and spiritual quest for truth. Through the mentorship and the spiritual direction of the Elders, he was guided back to the ceremonies of his people. The Elders helped him realize that First Nations people, despite enduring generations of profound suffering, scarcity and hardship as a result of being displaced from their original connection to the land and spiritual way of life, have survived because of the strength of the human spirit. The mentorship of the Elders provided Nii Gaani Aki Inini with inspiration, support, guidance and perspective on reaching a higher spiritual understanding, and a sense of the deep, sacred connection we have to the land. Since then he has traveled the world as a peace ambassador for many years.

I have learned to connect to back to nature in oneness from him and I hope by sharing his words you will begin to learn the joy and wonder of being connected as well.

I offer you his teachings near the end of this book to keep you encouraged and hopeful that we are shifting to a balance and harmony and he is getting the message out that as we respect the Earth, women and children we will also gain personal power to add our own part to Earth's healing. Dave's traditional name means 'Leading Earth Man' so what better chapter to put these teachings under then EARTH.

Sunrise Ceremony in Ontario
Excerpts - from my Journal
Thursday, July 27th 1995 – Evening Ceremony around the fire.

"This world we live in is not in harmony. Humans have forgotten about the Great Spirit and how Spirit is in everything. The spirit in us, in the animals, in plants and all living things from Mother Earth. All the while man is taking from her, raping her. Humans think material objects will bring ultimate happiness. But in reality it is nature and all she has to offer. We have to get back in touch with nature, with Mother Earth. We are her children, she provides for us even when we treat her with no respect. Somehow humans have grown apart from spirit.

When we were just spirit the creator asked us if we would like to walk Mother Earth, we all agreed. The only thing the Creator asked of us was not to forget our spirits. When we are born into this world we give a cry of joy that we made it. But as we are growing up there are so many negative things in our way that make us forget about our spirit. The indigenous people have been trying to show other humans the way they once lived and are starting to again. They are having visions and the spirits are telling them that we have to change our ways and start getting back to nature and all the spirits in nature."

We are outside, in the North country, around a sacred fire as David is giving his teachings over a period of days, it is dusk at this teaching and we are being eaten by mosquitoes, and we are all slapping at them.

David says to us: "There is a reason for everything on the Earth; before killing the mosquito asks its spirit what its reason is for being here. Humans don't try to understand anymore. If they don't understand something, they destroy it. He asks us to go into the trees tomorrow and feel Mother Earth. As we cleanse our bodies with the sweat lodge and fasting we open ourselves up more to hear spirit. We are giving up eating and drinking for a weekend for the spirits to help us, and they will reward us. It might not be this weekend but we will be rewarded." David explains when he talks about spirit he means it's not just seeing signs and visions, it is also about feeling. That is what spirit really means. It's about love. A very strong love *you can feel. Happiness is the Light, Caring, Sharing and Love. That is what all humans need and crave. But we have forgotten how to reach for the love. There is too much darkness in our world right now."*

David teaches us how to pray to the directions with our tobacco.

Friday, July 28th 2005

It rained throughout the night and we had to keep the fire burning day and night for the whole ceremony.

David begins the morning talk by saying we should say a prayer of thanks. We were blessed last night with the rain. It was a cleansing for us to start us on our journey. As he is speaking there is a distant sound of thunder. David says it is the Thunderbird. Thunder is the voice of God that we hear to give us proof of a Higher Being. Nobody is listening to God or praying anymore. The indigenous peoples have been having visions. The spirits are telling them that the Earth has to be cleansed. That there will come a time when the Thunderbird will use water and wind as a way of cleansing this land, and no human army or force will be able to fight against the Thunderbird. Spirit is calling people and they feel the pull to get back to nature and women are being affected by it the most. The spirits are drawing them in that direction.

A lot of people don't understand what is happening to them, but they should not be scared. Mother Earth is bringing the woman back to spirit, back to nature. Women are the bringers of life. Women are sacred. The world will become a much happier and loving place when we all join back together with Mother Earth and all her creations. But the dark side will always put tests in our way. It is easier to be led into temptation. So if we learn to not follow the dark side since our spirit always longs for love, we will be looked after when the world is made new again.

It's just like giving birth. First comes all the pain of labor, then the water comes, which is a cleansing, then the baby. If we pray for guidance or strength or whatever we need at the time to find love and tolerance, as long as we ask for it, we will get it. We come to pray instinctively when someone we love is ill or dying; we must learn to pray everyday and to thank the great spirit in the sky for everyday we are alive and to thank Mother Earth every day for all that she provides for us".

David finishes the morning ceremony with his pipe.

I am feeling very weepy and don't know why. One of the girls tells me to ask for a release so I can cry. Crying is a good thing she tells me, it is a cleansing. For me I was brought up with three brothers and was taught crying was wrong. That night we do a sweat lodge.

David started talking when all the stones were in and the door was closed. He said: "The sweat lodge represents the mother's womb and we are cleansing our bodies, thus making it easier for the spirits to communicate with us. Some people might be feeling very emotional and that was okay. Once again he told how mother earth is very sacred and how she takes care of her children. When the time comes when there is no water left on the surface that is drinkable, no matter what humans do to fix it with chemicals, she will show the humans that respect her and all of the world that are one with spirit where the water is. Mother earth is storing fresh water now beneath the Earth."

Saturday, July 29, 2005

I awoke crying and did not want to go to the morning ceremony and cry all the way through it, so I went into the woods instead. Later that morning I began menstruating. I was very upset, I thought of be careful what you pray for you just might get it. I prayed to be able to cry and it was only by getting my menstrual flow that I could release. I went to wait my turn to speak with David alone.

"I explained how I just got my cycle and it wasn't supposed to come until next week" He said, "It is just more proof how unbalanced Mother Earth is right now with something as dependable as a women's cycle which is to take place every 28 days: It is not so dependable anymore. He went on to say; "Women are very sacred because they are the givers of life. Women are to be honored. He said our moon time is a very powerful time for a woman. It affects the energy around her and of others.

When women live together nature brings their cycles at the same time, or if you were to live in a tribal community where ceremonies are done frequently as in the old ways. All women would be together and have their own ceremonies. A group of women on their cycle would overpower. David has seen dancers collapse from the energy being taken from them when there were women on their cycle in the same group. The vision quest ceremony is a very positive one, the sacred fire is positive, the sweats are positive. What is discharging out of a woman's body on her cycle may be viewed as negative in the sense it is all the old waste. That is why I need to sit surrounded by cedar as it holds in that energy. These are the laws of nature, man did not write the law. It was set in place since the beginning of time.

Women are blessed in the sense, as it is a cleansing of their bodies. Women are lucky they go through a cleansing every month. It is something that should be rejoiced about. And all humans should respect that. If men want to cleanse their bodies they have to do a piercing. Do not look upon it as a burden. Look upon your cycle as a time for giving life and a cleansing of the body. And remember how much closer woman is to mother earth in the sense that they are both givers of life and nurturers."

He then directed me, that I had to go get cedar and put it all around my tent. When I picked the cedar I was to sprinkle tobacco on the tree and to tell the spirit of the tree why I needed it. The spirit of the tree will be happy to give me what I need. He told me I could only leave my tent to go to the bathroom and I could only go back to the fire for the last feast because the ceremony would be over then. He told me I was blessed to be able to go to the sweat lodge last night.

The last night I was able to attend and we were finally having a meal. The first plateful of food was given to the fire as an offering. It was very hard to wait while all food was being brought out and then a plate made up for the fire, were all so hungry, but what a great feast we had and how thankful we were for it.

After we ate David stood up to talk. He told us: "*We should give another prayer of thanks to the Great Spirit, Mother Earth and all the spirits that helped lend their strength to us these past few days, in order to be able to find spirit ourselves. When we have found spirit we have to keep working at holding onto it. It is a feeling within us of love and warmth. Someone told me that they tingled all over and that is the spirit with them. People will try to take your spirit away from you. When you go home, that will be the real test, but try not to give in, pray everyday. Pray for strength, pray for other people who want to kill the spirit within you, ask that they be shown how to find their own spirit. It is especially hard in the city to remain peaceful and loving. Pray more. People will try to take the sparkle from your eyes. Try not to give into anger or to the darkness.*

The creator made four different colors of people. Each race has a certain gift that the creator gave to them. The white race has the gift of fire. That can easily be seen by all our inventions. The lights, t.v., phone, oven, computer etc. We have everything we need to survive. Mother Earth offers us the essentials. All our inventions are to make life easier, to have more time to pursue spirit. But when are we going to stop our inventions. We don't need anymore then we have now. But the people in the cities just keep coming up with bigger and better things. But at what cost to the Earth, and bigger and better for whose well-being.

It is a destructive path we are on with only a few people getting the message out that we are in serious need to stop destroying the planet. David tells us how he's been to the rainforest and how sad it is to see it disappearing. For we know what trees do for us, they give us oxygen to breathe. The government in this country is just as bad if not worse by looking down at other countries for destroying the forests but we do it all the time. He tells us a story that in Manitoba there is a mill. There is a type of tree they use but it had some kind of disease attacking these trees. With the government's approval they close off part of the forest and spray chemicals. Then they post a sign saying the forest has been sprayed, contaminated for a week. DO NOT ENTER. But meanwhile they've killed all the other plant life in that forest; the insects, the animals and birds that eat them.

David says an elder came up to him and asked; "When did the bears learn to read?", as they would be eating the berries from the forest.

This was all done in the name of progress. Humans have no care when they are on the road to progress. It doesn't matter what's in their path, be it mountain, river, animals or other humans. All our lives we are conditioned to think about the progress we must make now and in the future. We have to recondition our thinking to realize that everything we need to survive is provided to us by mother earth. We have to relax and enjoy each day at a time; stop rushing around and stop trying to fulfill the useless saying; "He who has the most wins" What do you win? You can't take it with you when your time has come. Then he tells us; "I don't want you to quit your jobs and go live off the land or anything drastic. We all need money; it can be used for good. If we didn't have money this weekend couldn't have taken place. We all needed transportation to get here. It's just a shame humans can't say okay, we have enough. Let's just sit back and enjoy the fruits of our labor and start to recognize other humans again. Recognize the spirit in people, in animals and start sharing the earth with everything that has a purpose for being here."

Sunday July 30 2005

This is the last day and we gather together around the fire before breakfast.

"David begins to tell us about the first time spirit came to him. He was a young boy and was very sick with pneumonia and the doctor said he couldn't do much. Then one night three grandfather spirits came as he slept. They told him not to fear them, they were there to help him get well. They told him to trust them and they instructed him and no matter what happened to trust them. They told David to take the beaver pelt from the other room and to place it on his chest so he did this but there was a lot of pain and he started moaning and yelling. His parents came into his room and David was clutching his chest and crying out in pain. His parents removed his hands to see what was wrong with his chest and found the beaver pelt.

Not knowing how or why he had it there they took it off him. In the morning David was well again. His fever had broken and he had no other symptoms. He told his parents about the grandfather spirits coming to visit him to make him well. His parents didn't believe him as they had been raised Christian and didn't know any of the old ways. He kept trying to tell them and everyone he met, but they just took it for childhood fantasies. As he got older he started having visions and he would tell people but they looked at him with disbelief in their eyes. So David stopped telling people of his experiences. But that is not what the spirits intended him to do when they came to him when he was sick. He was shown through visions that the higher being wanted him to teach the indigenous peoples the old ways.

As an adolescent he was shown how to talk to his people so they would listen and learn. Now he is being shown that he has to teach all humans, even with the disapproval of his own people. He feels an urgent need to inform people to stop harming Mother Earth. Humans have to start giving back, all they do is take. David says that people don't realize the seriousness of our situation, especially if they live in the city. Those who live in the city get caught up in the fast pace, there's not much time for yourself to sit and reflect. So with his closing he asks us all to take time to pray."

When I asked for permission to have his teachings in my book, Dave's assistant answered my email and said Dave would be honored. At the same time unbeknownst to me, Spirit was also moving through another woman to bring forth Dave's message in the form of a movie. This documentary film came out in the fall of 2007 and is called The 8th fire. I received the movie as a Christmas present, the movie presents two ancient prophecies the main one states, *"They will come to a fork in the road. One road will lead to materialism, and destruction…for almost all living creatures. The other road will lead to a Spiritual Way upon which the Native People will be standing. This path will lead to the lighting of the 8th fire, a period of eternal peace, harmony and a "New Earth" where the destruction of the past will be healed."* – Anishnabe Prophecy. The fire has been lit and continues to be lit at an elders gathering ever September and people from all races are invited to attend. Dave says: "When we light the Sacred Fire, we destroy our own intent. We invoke the spirit of prayer, as we call upon the spiritual realm to come and offer guidance and inspiration in our lives. …Our people refer to this as the rebirth of the earth because a rebirth would have to take place if we are going to prevent the destruction of our own planet."

The 8th Fire speaks about individuals from all different cultures who would gather collectively to seek greater advice and a vision that would lead to what is referred to as the "new people." The different cultures would share the uniqueness of each of their strengths and give teachings and knowledge to each other.

There are so many signs of hope, and for many people the New Earth has arrived and it is a wonder-filled experience. There is another prophecy in the movie about the new children who are known to the Native Tradition as "Warriors of the Rainbow". My personal experiences with Dave have been closely linked to helping children this is what I have experienced in the years he came to Ontario. I had a vision for children and golf because of Dave and it happened in 2002.

Journal excerpts- **November 17, 2002.**

Dave came to Ontario just before the war. He told us he was called by the world leaders of Peace to light a scared fire to burn for 40 days and 40 nights. The request came for Dave and the Elders to smoke their pipes in prayers for peace. The fire was started in Manitoba and he lit one with us in Ontario. He assured us there were many sacred fires all over the world burning at the same time. This was part of his teachings at that time.

"Help the children discover spirit. They need all the spiritual people helping them. They are our future. He cannot fathom all the children dying of disease and starvation while money is spent on destruction. Stop living in denial. We live in very challenging and exciting times because we are accelerating through spiritual growth that used to take yogis their whole life to achieve. We are now in an era of the time of truth. Look to the Native Spirituality for the proof of the strength of spirit to survive. The ancestors and the way they lived, sharing with everyone, loving everyone - that is why they invited the foreigners among them to share what they had. (We still celebrate this at Thanksgiving)

But they were only interested in the land and they could not understand the teachings. The sacred fire had to go underground. He was so grateful to be able to light one today and anytime."

This is what disturbs him the most about schools today, the lack of respect for the Indigenous people, that their children do not learn we are all brothers and sisters - everyone, even the people in Iraq, because we are all born from Mother Earth. The land, air, fire, water, we are a part of all these things. He likes to talk to the Grandmothers because he learns from them. He feels sorry for the youth. There are not many spiritual teachers teaching how sacred women are.

The girls are being shown the message that they are only good as marketable, not to bring out their dreams. We are all here to fulfill the Creator's dream of us. We as a society are not showing the girls how to connect with their inner beauty only the outer. Great Spirit has created a dream for each and every one of us. The dark forces need a balance. What can we do? Look to the Natives and how their spirituality has survived. Everything was taken from them, the white man tried to eliminate them. We need to get back to the land, we live only for comfort not for Creator, we love comfort more then the Creator."

Dave had a letter that he wrote for the Peace Leaders, which he shared with us that day. As he was reading it I was getting choked up, this is one of the times I did not record what was being said because spirit moved so strongly through me I had what can be termed as a kundalini awakening. Or what I termed an orgasm of the heart. I was opened up. I don't remember what his words were but I saw words in my own head. Brigham, Young and I saw a Golf Teacher named Sam Young and I was told to work with him. Now I knew Sam had a great reputation for his junior golf program because it was in our local paper quite often. When Dave finished talking he asked if anyone had anything to share. I said I did and it took a while to come out because I was crying, now my rational mind was judging me and couldn't figure out why I was crying.

I said to the group that I had a vision I am to work with children in regards to golf and I had asked for their prayers at the time to help me follow through with it. I then had to go outside, I couldn't be with people, and I couldn't be with sound. I went out into the woods and I had no thoughts in my head for the first time in my life. Unfortunately if you are not in a place like an ashram where you can just sit and meditate and have people are taking care of your daily needs like cooking it is not such a fun experience living in the daily grind.

I had a very hard time functioning when I went home. For the next 3 days I could not work, I could not even cook a meal. I was ungrounded, floating outside of my body, which many people thought sounded so cool, and which many yogic people aspire to. But it wasn't fun, from this experience I would only agree that it was cool if like I said you could be taken care of. I tried every way I could think of to ground myself and come back into my body but nothing helped but getting my menstrual cycle. This brought me fully back into my body. For the first time I really appreciated my monthly flow. My insight for this experience and others that I have gone through is that Grace descends down but that doesn't mean you live in the blissful state for long periods. We are part of the Earth and we are Spiritual Beings and the two can come together but then we can also fall back to sleep by living back in our conditioning.

After I was grounded, I did my best to working with Sam Young but it was not the right time. Even though I had the vision and I was pushing, it came but not my time but the universes time. It was three years later when I was blessed to work with junior golfers and to give them some of these steps to learn how to coach themselves to play great golf from the inside out. One summer I had an hour with 20 juniors from ages 8-18. It was definitely a challenge to convey my message in a way that each age group could grasp.

I ended up writing a story for them and giving it to them as a workbook. "Humble the Bumble bee and the Magical Golf Course." The next winter session I worked with a couple of the teenage girls who bloomed quicker in the semi-private class than in the summer with the mixed group of ages and genders. The emphasis of these sessions was more on confidence, trusting their bodies and to feel their swings.

I really love teaching golf as a metaphor for life and how the principles of yoga help for both. Helping children gain this advantage at an early age is so rewarding.

These teens had a good foundation of the swing mechanics and course management already they were very open and eager for the mind mastery aspect and really blossomed. It was such a delight to be with them and to pass along knowledge of confidence and loving themselves on and off the golf course.

I have noticed since Dave first urged us to help the children in 2002 that the role models for children are getting weaker not stronger except maybe in the sport of golf. What is the box, the T.V. showing? What they term reality shows, it's a part of all networks, but the damaging one for our daughters are ones like Pussy Cats and Coyote Ugly, it is all about what Dave's message was, the girls are being shown that they are only as valuable as how marketable or sexy they are, the focus is on the outer.

This isn't reality, but do the children know that? Thankfully there is a sport like golf that has wonderful role models for girls. This year, 2008 the LPGA Leader is Twenty six year old Lorena Ochoa who has worked hard to achieve her dreams. She is very down –to- earth and humble she is a great inspiration not only to Mexico but for all women and girls.

One of the last times I saw Dave in Ontario he was doing a talk at the University of Toronto and he was looking for other schools to go to. I was able to bring him to a very small school in the very small town in Alton. I will never forget this experience as long as I live. I had only seen him teach adults, but where he shines is teaching children. His being radiates Spirits love when he is teaching. To read my writings is not nearly as powerful as being in his presence. But I will try my best to convey it to you through this next example.

For the children he taught in a format using the teachings of the Seven Grandfathers. This was by using the animals and what they represented Love, Respect, Courage, Honesty, Wisdom, Humility and Truth. For example the beaver represents wisdom. The beaver uses wisdom by following its own nature, which it has been gifted as a wood chopper. If the beaver did not use its gifts its teeth would keep growing and eventually it would die because it would not be able to eat since its teeth would grow right through its bottom lip. Humans can learn from this wisdom to follow our own unique natures and gifts from the Creator. We all have our own unique gifts and talents and if we do not use them then a part of us dies inside. Dave teaches, " Our gifts do not belong to us, they belong to the world, to the people." Dave then asked the children what they liked to do as one way to help the children understand that may be they can already see a talent or gift they have been handed. Just through this one teaching he really conveyed the message they were special. This had a powerful effect on the children and with each illustration of the animals and their meaning the children felt more and more special.

At the end when he was asking for questions he was getting asked to speak in his native tongue a lot. Then one little girl put up her hand, and I will never forget what she had to say. Dave said "yes" She put both hands in together in front of her heart and with such emotion said to Dave "you are such a good man," I was standing in the front of the children with Dave and the Love that passed with this child's words was so strong it was like a ripple I could almost see that passed towards Dave. Dave said "thank you, you made my day". But what the child didn't know was that she made my day as well! Just by being the observer I could feel the love so strong and pure I have never forgotten it. I also saw how impressed all of the children were by Dave because when they were asked if they would like to be in a Picture with Dave.

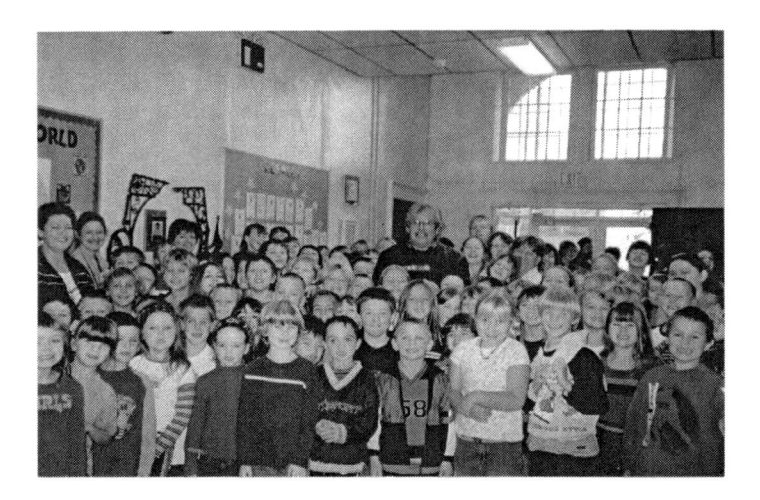

The kids moved in so fast to circle around him, I have never witnessed anything like that before It was like he was a magnet and they were pieces of metal attaching themselves.

Yes, there are many who are in tune with what really matters, and they are making a difference but we obviously need to set a better role model for the girls. There are many children coming to help us; Indigo, Crystal, Rainbow, but many get just as lost as us with the T.V. viewing of non-stop shows that are all beginning to look like the sexual music videos. Once again I refer to the prophecy in the Movie the 8th fire we are living in the time of the "Warriors of the Rainbow," they are here among us now.

They are system busters to help heal our world, one of the areas they are here to break down is the old school system, this is a bad program we have been fed and these children recognize this and what is happening to them, they are getting put on drugs like Ritolin so they will sit still. Maybe they are not supposed to sit and listen but be listened to. Maybe they need to be outside in Nature learning from Mother Earth.

Once children used to play outside all the time, the school program could be balanced with being out in nature. I live near three schools and I was concerned at first it may be a noisy neighborhood but all the kids are inside. Where is the balance of being indoors and outdoors. If we can bring them to the golf course they are outside for hours. Maybe we need more golf courses designed for children and families. Golf is a great tool to learn integrity and honesty; no other sport allows you to call a penalty on yourself. Children are honest little beings until we begin to train them what society expects, in other words brain washing. We can learn from them, that honesty may disrupt things, but in the end it would be a lot healthier place for all of us to live. The wonderful thing about children is they can help bring out our inner child, help us to lighten up, and help us to stay young at heart.

One final piece I have discovered through the native path is one of the Nature's Laws, the Law of Giving and Receiving. The First Nations embrace this principle with their potlatch or give-a-way ceremonies. I have been told of give-a ways of entire house contents only to have the house fill up again with contents from others the same day. The lesson from nature is the giving does not always come back from the same receiver but from many sources. The underlying message here is of pure trust in nature and since we are connected it is a part of our nature, we are generous beings.

Now, what I find interesting is Golf is such a great sport in following this Natural Law. Golf gives back generously, we see this throughout the sport, from the touring Pro's playing for charity events to charity's themselves trying to raise money and finding much success by holding Golf Tournaments. Do you suppose it is because it is a game that is played upon Mother Earth for hours? She has had a strong influence on golfers, without people even being aware of it. The flip side of the coin to Greed is Generosity. Giving is a very simple act and many can attest to the fact that if you give with the right intent you receive seven fold.

One way to give back to our Mother Earth is by fasting, for thousands of years, many cultures around the world fasted for purification and to give of themselves for the greater good. More and more people today are again realizing the benefits of fasting.

I personally do not think it is necessary to fast for many days at a time it can be a simple as one day, four times a year with the change of the seasons. The following benefits come from Dave Courchene Jr. and his Turtle Lodge teachings:

- Fasting gives our bodies and the Earth a rest and allows us to cleanse, de toxify and heal. Historically, people lived on a sparse diet free from pesticides, food additives, drugs and toxins. Today we consume more toxic substances than all the generations before us. Levels of built-up lead in our bones can be 200 times greater compared to those excavated 2000 years ago. Children today are born with toxic blood. Through air, water, food and even mother's milk there is absorption of thousands of toxins and chemicals that saturate the environment. These toxins have affected the Earth and our bodies.

• Fasting overhauls the respiratory, circulatory, digestive and urinary systems. It helps destroy all the impurities of the body and all sorts of poisons. It eliminates uric acid deposits.

• Fasting begins to help us reach a higher level of understanding life and our connec ion to the Earth. We have arrived at a point in our evolution that we must stop and look at where we are going as humanity. Is our current course one of sustainability? Going on a fast helps bring us to a STOP to consider our future. We need to consider our humanity. We need to consider what we are doing to ourselves. We need to consider what we are doing to the land.
• Fasting is a way of showing love for our children. We need to consid
er our children's future. Our children are our future. What we do to the Earth we do to our children and future generations. When we take from the Earth we are taking from our children's legacy. When we give to the Earth and to ourselves through the act of Fasting, we are investing in our children. We need to put our children back into the center of our lives.

• Fasting helps rebalance us and reconnect us to the land. Obesity and other health problems are symptoms of our imbalance and disconnection, and also reflect the amount of toxins and chemicals that have been introduced into the natural food chain.

• Fasting will support the realization of how life is all related and connected to the Earth, and could bring in a new paradigm of thinking about our values and behavior.

Goddess Gaia representing the Back Nine

Hole 16 – Sacred Play

Playing with a joyful attitude is one of the best ways to know if you are playing in a sacred way. A playful attitude enhances everything; play enhances golf, play enhances yoga and of course play enhances life. My first yoga book that I ever did yoga from was Richard Hittlemans 28 days of yoga. His description said all are parts are disjointed. For example the body may want to rest, the mind wants to be working on problem solving and the spirit wants to play. The confusion ends when all parts are in harmony. Not many people I have taught over the years are in harmony, especially playing golf. When you find your authentic self, harmony, peace and happiness are the end result. The golf book by *Steven Pressfield, 'The Legend of Bagger Vance'*, tells a story that is a metaphor about the authentic swing being the analogy for the authentic self.

If we are going back in nature to play, whether on the golf course or in some other way, it is time we go back with a greater sense of awareness, respect and responsibility to ourselves, the earth and all her children, human or otherwise. Let's make it deep, make it real, we and the earth are worth it.

Think about how children learn, by playing games, this does not stop ever, but we view ourselves as adults and we need to be serious now so many don't think about playing in terms of learning. Golfers are very lucky to continue to learn by playing. Golf, just like life, is filled with paradoxes and a lot of the time we only need to change our perception. We have been taught that sand and water are seen as obstacles on the golf course. Another way to view them is an opportunity to play better golf. If we land in the sand, we can say "Oh, here is an opportunity to practice with my wedge."

A great way to begin your day on the golf course is to bow to Mother Earth. This way we humble ourselves before her to teach us the lessons for the day. In Yoga there is a word 'Namaste' which means, *"The divine in me recognizes the divine in you."* This is a similar act that the opponents use in Martial Arts, bowing to each other before they begin. We can use the Yoga Mudra pose with or without a golf club. To others it just looks like a pre-game stretch but for Golfing Goddesses it is the beginning of sacred play. We bow forward and silently say "Namaste" to Mother Earth, although we don't view her as an opponent like in Martial arts, but our teacher and playing guide.

Come, Be Golfing Goddesses!

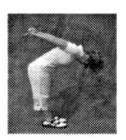

One of the best recourses I have used for years is a book by Ted Andrews called- 'Animal Speaks' I first used it for messages in my life and then in golf as a way to understand my connectedness with everything living upon Gaia. It helped me recognize that all answers do lie within but sometimes as humans can't see the forest through the trees. That is because we are too close to our problems and our minds can chew and chew over a subject and do not always give us the best answer that our inner core can. Ted's book has helped me to ask Mother Earth to reveal an animal while playing so I can see what I lesson I need in my life at the moment. All animals have a message (or medicine) and this can be learned by examining their characteristics and living patterns. The book 'Animal Speaks' gives readers an in depth look into each animal, bird, insect, even trees and flowers to help people recognize there are energies that can influence everything and we can learn from these sources.

In many characteristics of the meaning of each animal or bird it relates how it can help in everyday life and some even give you questions to ponder. Learning through the animals will not only connect you deeper to nature but will help you acquire a new belief system to replace old out molded ones. Why would we want to do this? Because if you are suffering from your old beliefs you will keep attracting the same scenario's over and over. I heard a story once that describes how our choices attract to us our beliefs, and it may help you move away from pain and towards wholeness and harmony.

Illustration-
Once long ago a man approached a village and he was greeted by the gatekeeper. He asked the gatekeeper what the kind of people lived in this village. The gatekeeper replied, "What were the people like where you came from?" And the man answered that the people were unkind, rude and selfish and the gatekeeper said, " I'm sorry to say you will find the same kind of people here." Another day passed and another traveler came to the village and asked the gatekeeper the same question. "Good man, I was hoping you could tell me about the people of this village. What are they like?"

The Gatekeeper responded with the same question he asked the first man. "What were the people like where you came from?" "Oh," the man said, "They were wonderful, very kind, thoughtful and generous, I hated to leave but I have an opportunity to work in this village for higher pay." The gatekeeper assured him he would find the same kind of folk in this village.'

Come, Be Golfing Goddesses!

Think about this story in the terms of someone wanting to join a country club and asking the same questions and giving the same answers. This story is a great example of how our choices in seeing the world is a mirror and reflects back to us what we believe. Now we can change that belief and the outer world will change as well.

I believe as women if we can spend, as much time playing upon Gaia, the faster the end result to our authentic selves will occur. In today's fast paced society when I say this to the women I know I usually get the same response," I don't have time". It is easy to understand as women are multitaskers without even trying. I have spent many years as a single parent, running a household, being mother and father, a cook, a handy woman and owning and operating a yoga studio at the same time. I know there is little energy and time left at the end of the day. In yoga there is a saying, "You slow down to speed up". What this means essentially is when you are moving at a mile a minute you can't hear the voice of spirit who can direct you to make one action correctly instead of doing five incorrectly.

I remember last year my daughter telling me she worked 14 hours one day and didn't get anything done. In her words, "I am so frustrated." So of course I recommended a day off to refresh and to gain a new perspective. Being in nature is one of the best places to soothe the soul and become creative once more. Now when suggest spending time in nature not many people, men or women, would just go out for four hours. It is almost unheard of in these busy days of ours. But think about it; that's what it usually takes to play 18 holes of golf. Again the golf course is a perfect place to take a time out. Being in nature and the beauty of the courses is like a balm on the mind and emotions.

Here's a technique to try ... before you arrive at the course, bring to mind a problem you need a solution for and firmly state to yourself as soon as you step onto the course you will not let your mind chew it over and over while you are playing. As soon as you step off the course, if it wants to come back to the forefront of your mind again, fine. By letting it go you will find the solution comes easily. It might not be as soon as you walk off the course but be aware; it could be a song you hear on the way home, a show on TV. or a phone call with a friend.

Don't be attached to how it comes. Be open and confident it will and in the best possible manner. Why? Because you are taking a time-out for the left-brain, which is the problem solver and you are creating space for the right brain, the creative side, a chance to work on the solution. When you give directions to yourself like that you allow your powerful subconscious mind to go to work on your behalf. Usually when we are trying to figure something out with our conscious mind we limit ourselves. We allow the wise part of ourselves the reigns. We can get something even better than we thought. We can train ourselves to put ourselves first when we are at the end of our rope. We need to fill up our wells so it's not crap we're giving to family and friends; its patience and tolerance. To be able to smile and not scream or release heavy sighs, which incidentally is just the body's way of releasing the screams we are afraid to let out.

I learned this first hand as a child myself, then as a mother, and finally by teaching other mothers. You see, I was first introduced to yoga through my mother in the 1970's when I was a pre-teen. Throughout my childhood my mother was always on edge and screaming at my brothers and me. When she began yoga she totally transformed into a calm and patient woman. She seemed more loving, I know she loved us but the stress covered it up so her actions didn't portray this. I would go with her to some classes, which were so different in those days. The ladies wore leotards and tights and we brought sleeping bags to do the yoga on.

But it wasn't the physical aspects that stayed with me it was how calm my mother became that impressed me which I now know is the result of the union, the joining together of the mind/body/spirit. The funny thing is how I became my mother when my children were young, even though she had more patience with us, as we grew older. The way she raised us when we were young is what I was emulating to my kids. I was very aware of how low my tolerance level was so I said, "Mom I need your yoga books." My outlook changed like I hoped it would; I fell in love with yoga and became a certified teacher myself.

The feedback over the years from my students has been so rewarding. I have even received a picture from one of my student's daughters whom I had never met, but the love her mother received in class came home to her. Over and over my students have said the families can see the benefits and my students aren't aware of any changes. If some took a season off they were highly encouraged to go back to yoga by their families.

It becomes a win/win for everyone. Now to add a spiritual program to golf is the highest winning combination that leads to the path of the heart and to come back to unconditional love that is all around us. Look to the elements in the four directions they provide to us unconditionally. A great contemplation to do is the energy of the sun and how it provides, in the providing it does not judge. It shines on everything unconditionally everything is equal to the Sun. The trees, ocean, animals, and every color of plant and human life, we are beings under one Sun. I am so grateful for the help of the Goddess over the years we have a Loving relationship and I have seen her transform many others to live magical lives. Once women surrender to the divine feminine energy and begin to witness for themselves that their own consciousness makes a difference they will start to pay more attention to it and use it more wisely.

The more we begin to send thoughts of Love and Gratitude to the golf courses and even driving ranges, the more we are doing our part in healing this planet. This is because many of these areas of mother earth are places that are covered with heavy dense energy. They have been areas that are allowed to be dumping grounds of golfer's negative thoughts and energy. The earth has absorbed years and years of anger and frustration from golfers. Just imagine how much gratitude games will help lift the heavy energy that surrounds most golf courses this raised energy will effect everyone consciously and unconsciously.

Now conversely many people who go away on golf retreats are in gratitude already and may not realize this is why they like to get away because the golfing seems more fun, easy and relaxed.

The inspiration for Gratitude Games came from one of my students whom I mentioned as being my earth angel, under the theme Intuition. Diane Pitcher has been a wonderful support and many times she has not been aware of this fact. I would like to share Diane's story of a tragedy that has befallen upon her life, and how she can be an inspiration when any bad golf games get you down.

Diane's story of finding her hero within

"Being an avid golfer, you can imagine my devastation when approximately two years ago I discovered I had to be on oxygen 24 hours a day for the rest of my life.

It really all began in the spring of 2006. I was visiting friends in Connecticut and found myself very tired and out of breath all of the time; not really being able to do very much. This continued until the fall when I just could not take it anymore and had a friend take me to the Hospital. They discovered my blood oxygen level was very low because I developed Pulmonary Fibrosis and my only alternative was the oxygen. Now I am dealing with anger and resentment over the fact that I would not have Pulmonary Fibrosis if I had not been given an antibiotic for a urinary tract infection to take over a lengthy period. In rare cases the antibiotic causes Pulmonary Fibrosis - I was one of those rare cases. So some days are better than others and I try to live the good ones to the fullest. I also have to deal with people who think because I am attached to an oxygen cylinder that I am a different person. They don't realize that I am the same person inside.

Basically I felt my life was over, and some days it really felt that way. Other days were better. I have fought every step of the way. I am certainly not the person I used to be. Last year for approximately nine months I had a trainer to help get myself back into shape and to help strengthen my upper body for my golf swing.

I also do gentle fitness and aerobic classes at a nearby senior centre.

A year ago I moved into a senior residence where my meals are prepared and I get help with cleaning and laundry. I am then able to use my energy on things I enjoy

doing. I am still a member at Oakville, but only a Social Member, which allows me to play a few times a month with a playing member. I sometimes play at other courses, but didn't do that this year, 2008.

I have been out golfing about 5 times - usually play up onto the green and then have someone pick up my ball. It is difficult to walk from the cart over to the green to putt - takes a lot of my breath away. Anyway a little is better than not at all.

"I asked her why she loved Golf?" Now, why I love the game. There are many reasons. The camaraderie, fresh air and exercise golf is a game you can play at any age, and by yourself if necessary. When I play I am only competing with myself.

I love the feeling of peace and contentment when I am on the course. I really don't know how to explain the way I feel when driving down the lush green fairway getting ready to hit the next shot.

I have to tell you that I played last Tuesday and I still have my game. Had some really good shots and the good ones keep you coming back again and again."

Take care,
With love and positive vibes,
Diane Pitcher

I can imagine how inspiring she would be to other players. It is very noble of her to continue playing and doing the best she can on her good days.

More inspiring Women Golfers

While teaching Yoga for Golf the summer /08 a woman in the class was telling me how inspired she is with the older members at her golf and country club; I thought her story would make a great addition to this book so I met with her and another woman from the club over tea. This meeting was intended as a first interview before being introduced to the rest of the members.

Though after the first meeting I felt I gained enough information to help encourage other women that there is no reason they can't continue to play all their lives.

I was told there are quite a few women in their late 70's and into their 80's and they are still competing and winning tournaments because of the handicap system. These are women who would be considered the crones in the Goddess Tradition, Grandmothers in the Native tradition and wise women to my way of thinking.

Without any labels however, they are just girlfriends getting together and are happening to stay young through Golf. They are a source of inspiration to the members since many still walk the hilly golf course, play several times a week and still play from the white tees!

When I asked the two what they loved about golf? I was told, *"how they love being out in nature and improving themselves. They expressed feeling very fortunate to belong to a great club with a great course to play upon and how like them the members live and breathe golf."*

They went on to described, *"feeling blessed to be living a golfing lifestyle which has allowed them to gain friendships for life."*

This is when the spark of enthusiasm took over while describing the friendships and all the support for one another, from one another. The fond memories of the golf trips they take together that brings forth a closer bond. The healthy outlook they notice the older members have and their sense of humor about getting on in years.

If for health reasons some women can't play any more they still go to the club to socialize and play bridge. They are part of a community that has imbedded in it all the grace from years of battle, play and character building inherent within the game.

As the meeting came to a close these two women did express some sadness that they do not see younger women golfers play competitively these days. They understand that it is a time factor however they would like them to know that they really like to play with the younger women. I personally think it could be beneficial for both ages, I was told one reason these women liked to play with the younger generation is because it keeps them sharp. I imagine the younger women could benefit since the older members have so much nurturing and wisdom to give. Not only these grandmothers but all grandmothers have stories that our society can benefit from if only we could accept their history/ her story with humility and curiosity.

Chapter 8

Artemis – Greek Earth Goddess Grounding and Intention

Myth- *An Earth Goddess who hunted daily in a chariot drawn by stags with golden antlers, she was the mistress and protector of animals. In neglecting their livestock, mortals offended the goddess. Artemis also enjoyed dancing and singing and the company of a retinue of nymphs. In Greek art, she was often pictured flanked by the wild beasts she hunted. She brought prosperity and long life to mortals she favored.*

-Eric Chaline

Poem to Artemis
I am who I am
and I know who I am
I can take care of myself
under all circumstances
and I can let others care for me
I can choose
There is no authority
higher than my own
my powers of discernment are finely honed
I am autonomous
I am free from the influence
of others' opinions
I am able to separate
that which needs separation
so a clear decision
can be reached
I think for myself
I set my sights
and aim by bow
my arrows always find their mark

The Mythology

Artemis (pronounced *ar'teh-mis*), another multidimensional Goddess reduced by the Greeks to the domain of moon, virgin, huntress, and childbirth, really represented the Feminine in all her aspects. She was the huntress who protected animals and the virgin (whole and complete unto herself) who made love in the woods. When Artemis was a little girl, Zeus, her father, wanted to give her a gift and asked her what she wanted. The Goddess replied: "I want to run forever wild and free with my hounds in the woods and never, ever marry."

The Lessons of this Goddess

Artemis has shot her arrow of selfhood in your life to help you focus on yourself. Have you been too much at the service of others without making sure you get what you need for yourself? Has it been too long since you had time to yourself or a space of your own? Do the boundaries of your selfhood seem blurred and indistinct? Do you feel you have no right to a self of your own, but must always be thinking of others, putting their needs first, until you don't know who you are or what you want? Now is the time to come into yourself. Now is the time to pay attention to the whispering voices of your own needs. Now is the time to take yourself back and celebrate and strengthen who you are. The Goddess says that wholeness is nurtured when you honor, respect, and give time to yourself. She also asks how can you expect to hit any targets if you don't have self from which to shoot?

http://angelfire.com/va/goddesses/atemis/html

Goddess Artemis representing the Front Nine

Hole 8 - Grounding

Artemis is the Goddess with whom I resonated the most with while growing up. I was a tomboy in my youth and I, like her would love roam wild and free in the woods. She is the representation I associated with in fairy tales. Being surrounded by the animals, the adventures of finding a witches house in the woods was more appealing to me then finding Prince Charming. Now that I am beginning to live with a more open heart, I am noticing the animals are not so afraid of me. They come closer all the time and it fills me with such wonder and gratitude. With my heart filled with gratitude I walk even lighter upon the Earth. I read once that Artemis can be called upon to help us Walk our Soul Walk. This is a great image for me while playing I see myself as 'walking the soul walk' on the courses.

In India the feet are said to represent the most sacred part of the body. Indian disciples bow down and touch the guru's feet, their most sacred part. Our feet are the hands that touch the Earth. They represent the foundation, the seat of understanding. The light heartedness of viewing our golf as a soul walk helps our footsteps become lighter, which helps mother earth raise her vibrations.

What needs to come first respecting our bodies or respecting the earth's body?

I would like to share what I wrote many years ago about how I learned to respect my body through Hatha yoga.

This piece is written in the same vein as "Everything I learned about life I learned in kindergarten", I titled it: <u>Everything I learned about my body I learned from yoga</u>

1. I expect perfection from it or life.
2. I've learned that my body has its own unique language there are different signals for different experiences.
3. If I don't listen to the sublet messages from my body the signals get louder and louder until I am forced to listen.
4. My body is my friend.
5. The inside of my body is like a well functioning machine, with many

systems that work automatically.
6. I need to keep my body relaxed for my mind to be creative.
7. Yoga poses help my body and mind release emotional build up.
8. Through yoga I've learned that how my mind thinks, my body responds and any disease I get was first produced by my thoughts.
9. As I keep my body strong and flexible I can stay focused longer without having distractions from aches and pains.
10. Last but not least I finally understand the cliché "you are what you eat". If I eat too much sugar and junk food my body is heavy and sluggish and it is harder to do my yoga.

What do we learn from the Earth element and our bodies? The most important is being grounded. Why the need to ground ourselves? Because we are part of this earth, we need to function here we need to balance the spiritual and the physical to do our soul's work. It is important to find our foundation, our roots. When we are ungrounded we are spacey, living in our heads, not our bodies. We will learn to get back in touch with how it feels to be fully connected inside ourselves. The pay off is, we make firm clear decisions, with focus and ease. We also manifest our dreams when we are grounded, they become a reality. Most of the time it is only by attending yoga classes that people truly experience what it is like to be grounded there is no real understanding of what the word means until they experience it for themselves.

I hope to be able to offer you the concept even if it is only a little for your body until I come out with a DVD that will reveal the feeling more intensely. I learned the following grounding technique years ago from a friend and then I add my own twist of combining affirmations with it – this is for home practice only.

Turkish Grounding

Stand with legs hip distance apart. Now do some pumps for about one minute. (You may find you want to skip this part at first and go directly to # 1).Pumps would be similar to lying down pelvic tilts except your standing. Try and imagine the golden core at the center of the earth and you are drawing up that energy into your belly to energize your third chakra, your inner sun.

Come, Be Golfing Goddesses!

1. Take your hands and place on top of forehead, Inhale and bring hands down to belly. Exhale and bend forward.

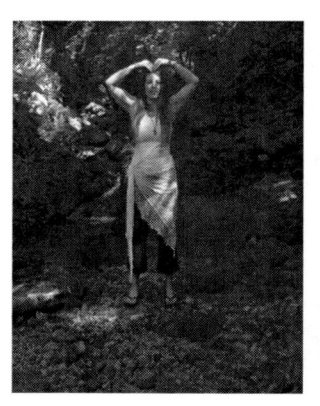

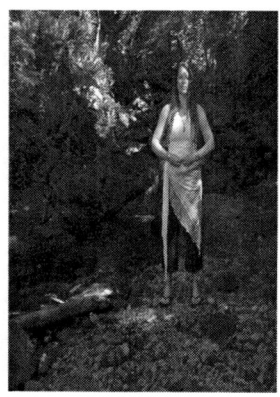

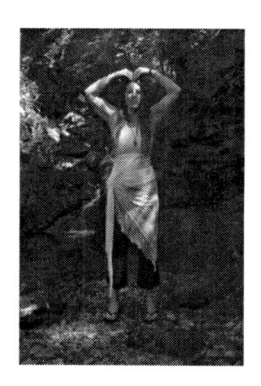

2. Inhale arms up overhead and exhale down to toes for two more times.

3. Inhale up for a the third time, exhale hands to hips.

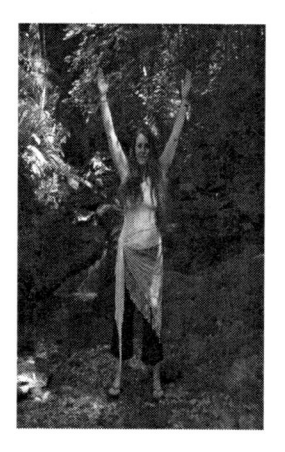

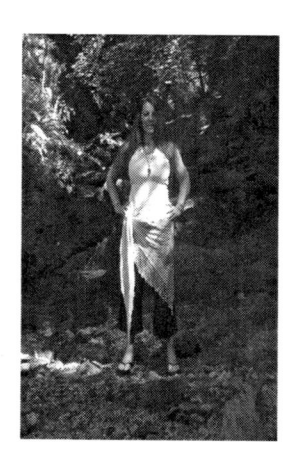

Come, Be Golfing Goddesses!

4. Rotate right hip in a circle three times, then rotate left hip three times

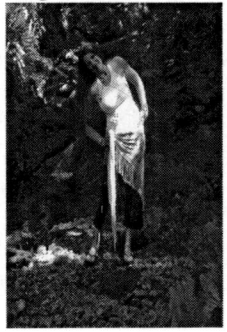

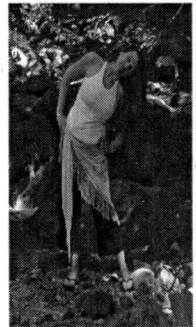

5. a) Place hands on low back

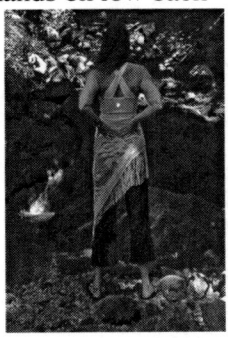

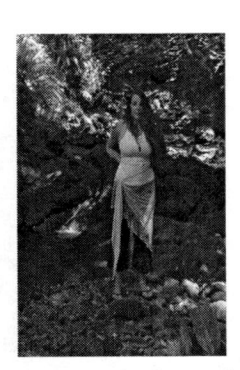

5. b) inhale while simultaneously brushing hands down the back of the legs to your feet,

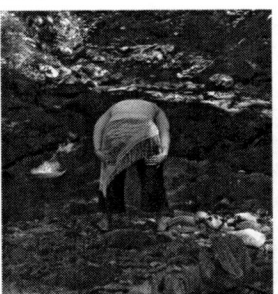

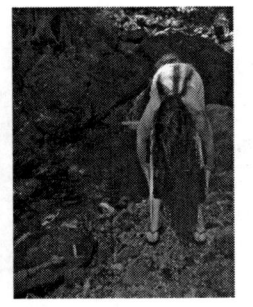

Come, Be Golfing Goddesses!

5. c) Than exhale, sliding hands up the front of the legs

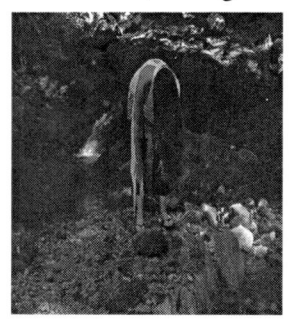

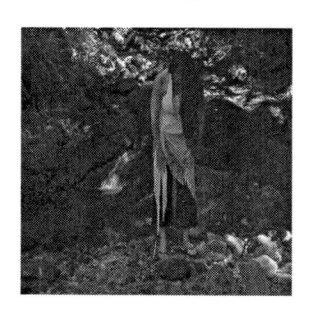

Repeat 2 more times.

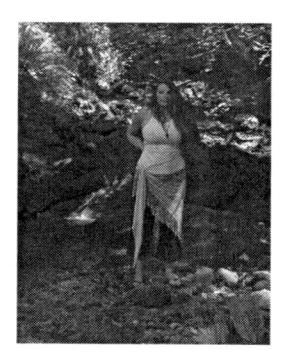

5. d) bring hands to belly

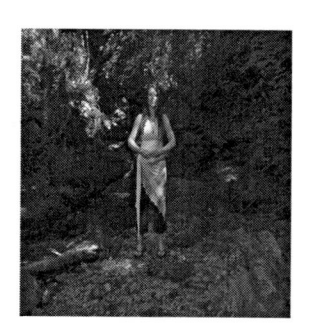

6 a). Inhale as you brush hands down the inside of the legs to the feet,

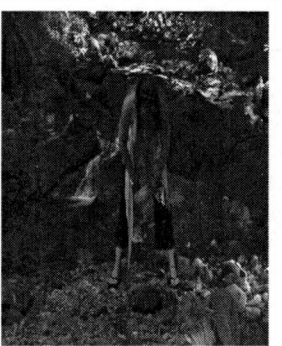

6 b). Exhale and you bring the hands up the outside of the legs resting hands back to the belly. Repeat 2 more times.

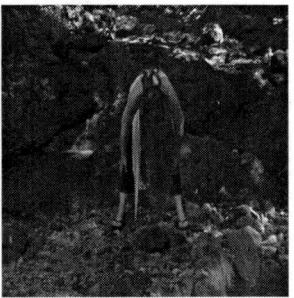

7. Bring hands to your heart center,

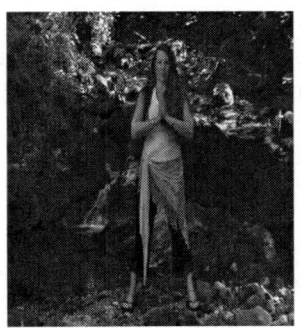

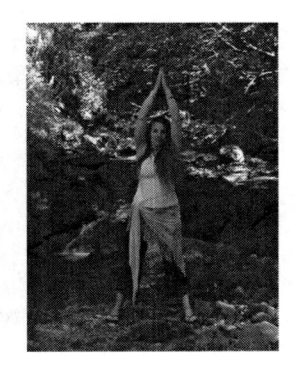

arms up overhead and

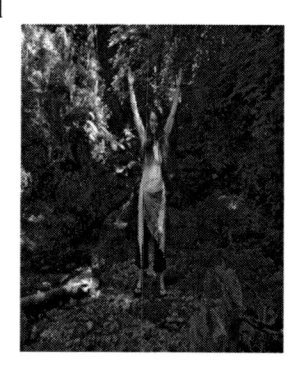

Exhale in a circle back to heart center.

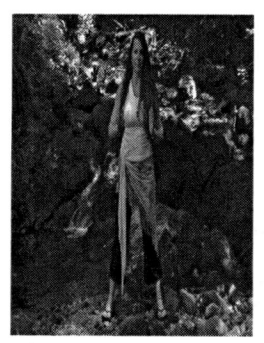

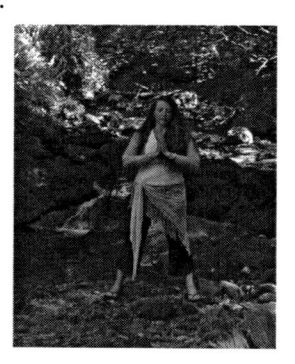

Repeat two times.

Grounding Pose
Hold the last position and tune into your body; consciously let your body weight drop down into the legs and feet.
REPEAT THE WHOLE SQUENCE TWO MORE TIMES, with each check in at the end feel more and more connected to the ground beneath you. Allow yourself to sink into it.

Affirmations with grounding pose.
After the hips circles we begin the affirmations. The first position as the hands are sliding down the back of the legs repeat is „I DESERVE', then repeat any affirmation as the hands are sliding up the front of the legs. For a total of 3 x's Moving on to the next movement the words are „I AM WORTHY' as you bring the hands on the inside of the legs, then repeat the affirmation as the hands move up the outside of the legs. 3x's in total.

When the hands are at the heart center Repeat the words "I ACCEPT' as you raise hands then repeat the affirmation as you circle the arms down around the body. Repeat 3 xs. The affirmations could be all the Goddesses attributes in this book or anything else you desire to bring into form.

The whole procedure from step one is repeated two more times. Once you become familiar with this grounding technique you will be able to check to see how you feel at the beginning and then at the end. You will find your feet much more planted into the floor. It's as if all your body weight drops to your legs and feet.

The fun part happens when you add affirmations to this grounding technique. What you desire can be brought about much quicker when used this way. For example, you may want to begin with the affirmation "I am a Golf Goddess!" The affirmations would be used from step five to step seven.

- The wording for step five would be "I deserve" as you bring the hands down the back of the legs and saying, "to be a Golf Goddess" as you bring the hands up the front of the legs.
- The wording for step six would be, "I am worthy" as you bring the hands down the inside of the legs, then saying, "of being a Golf Goddess" as you bring the hands up the outside of the legs.
- The wording for step seven would be, "I accept" as you bring the arms overhead, and then as the arms come down in a circle you state, "I am a Golf Goddess."

Other affirmations you may want to use are, trust, I deserve trust, I am worthy of trust, I accept trust or you can try it with confidence, happiness, money or anything else you desire." This exercise can be used for anything you want in your life; it doesn't have to apply specifically for golf. If you need more wealth, success or love in your life just pick what you need and do the same phrase for a time being. Wait and be aware of the subconscious going to work to bring you what you want. Watch for the signs, become excited when you see the evidence and that you will move towards the next phase of the intention that brings the pearls of wisdom closer to you.

Goddess Artemis representing the Back Nine

Hole 17 - Intention

"Whatever you vividly imagine, ardently desire, sincerely believe, and enthusiastically act upon…must inevitably come to pass!"
–Paul J. Meyer

    I have seen for myself and for many of my students when we begin to put forth our intentions to the Universe, the Universe answers back in the form of meaningful coincidences. There is the feeling of excitement when this happens. Then when my students are left on there own without the classes to keep the momentum going, the excitement fades and then the coincidences seem to go stale.

    This is where the discipline of using all the other steps before comes back into play. If you have been doing the steps and stopped, I encourage you to begin again. It doesn't take as long to get back into the flow of effortlessness. Let us recap what those steps are. We want to control the thought-waves in our mind by first replacing any doubt or fear that may have started to become dominate over the positive thoughts, so we go back to the affirmations. From the affirmations the next step is to work on a small goal. Success breeds success. We may still have one big goal for the year or for our career. But when we see smaller goals come to pass it leads to confidence knowing the big ones are on there way. We then detach from the outcome, we live confidently in the Great Mystery to bring us our goals in the right time and manner. Realize that goals are a way of beginning the collaboration with the Universe or your sub-conscious mind for self- direction helping to pointing yourself in the direction you want to go with your golf and life.

    Now we come to intention, which I have found is a more concentrated and collaboration with the flow. More one pointed. You are not in a wishful state anymore. When you are using intentions, you KNOW what you desire will come to pass. You demand it in the present tense, you feel worthy of receiving. YOU become a magnet because you put forth more energy, more desire for what you want. The next thing you know, an idea comes out of the blue on the steps to take to bring you towards your intended desire. This has happened while writing this book; I have talked quite a bit about getting a hole-in-one while I taught a few classes at a driving range this summer/08 my partner simultaneously took golf lessons. He then went on to make two holes in one. The first one I blogged about in August on the Yoga for Golf blog, (the address is at the back of the book). Now the powerful thing that happened in the game which I did not blog about and still haven't because I wanted to save it for this book; Is when my partner and I went to play his first golf game he mentioned he wasn't playing very well and I said, "you are just getting warmed up". Then I remembered our basketball and badminton games and how this year we were joking around and called in the Goddess Nike and the swoosh to help us. We had amazing effortless results, so as we were waiting to tee off at the 6th hole I said "call in the Goddess Nike." He did without question he trusted completely that the energy would help him because we have seen it happen before.

When it was his turn to hit tee-off his first ball drippled to the right. I told him I would give him a Mulligan, the next ball did the exact same thing. I said, "okay this can be another Mulligan but you wouldn't get this with any other players" and then the third shot was a *hole- in- one*. We were so happy the group behind us clapped as we walked up to see if it was really in the hole and the group in front a fellow asked what is your technique and Paulo said "Two Mulligans" but it was calling in the Goddess Nike! I'll tell you why I am so sure that it was this technique because he did it again!

The driving range I worked at had just put in mini-putting and we played a game a week after we went golfing. Now I don't know what it is called when you are mini-putting and you get it in the hole in one shot. But this is what happened. The hole was up hill with a big rock at the top of the hill the green went up and the hole was on the far left of the green. Paulo hit the first couple of balls right off the green trying to get it up hill. I said, "call in the Goddess Nike" he said "Oh yea" and the next shot went up the hill hit the side bank and went right in the hole. Again with the Mulligans first, but he stayed relaxed, surrendered to Nike and let that energy of victory move through him for his second hole- in-one after calling in the Goddess for help.

We have not been out to play another game but if he gets more holes-in-one I will encourage him to write a book on' Golfing God's a man's perspective from playing in the female vibe. I did not add Nike to this book, I see I don't really need to because she has been called forth into our dimension for many years, even if people do so unknowingly. What I know of Nike is that she is a Greek Goddess of Victory and on her heels are wings that the company Nike have used as a swoosh symbol. We can all attest to the fact that this company has been successful. And people who have Nike as their sponsors generally have success as well, especially if they are not coming from their ego selves. I love the symbolism of Tiger wearing the Nike hat that has the word ONE on the side of it. What I think is interesting is that Tiger Woods really is one with all four races on the medicine wheel. He has a mix of Afro-American, Asian, Caucasian and Native American heritage although he only recognizes two parts of his heritage.

Since I spent much of the spring and summer this year volunteering for The 8th Fire Movie and Ceremonies I unintentionally called forth the number 8. I had the final screening with Elder Dave Courchene come back to B.C. on 8.8.08. I was writing the numbers over and over again in emails, flyers and posters. I was involved with the energies or vibration of the number eight and what happened is the energy of this number came back to me and taught me about itself.

We can be involved with anything we put our attention on, everything is energy, it just vibrates differently so it shows up differently, and there is intelligence in everything. One thing I learned from this number is the next step to learning the meaning from the First Nations elders who teach, be careful what you put into your circle. I have come to learn there is more than just one circle for giving and receiving when we use intentions it is a giving process and we receive from another circle which then resembles the figure eight. Our thoughts, words, and actions go into the circle we are living in, the next circle is the infinite intelligence that hears and brings it back the energies closer to us. Using the power of intention helps the energy to spin with more intensity when we can understand

Once you understand that absolutely every infinite thing we know about and (don't know about) is energy in motion. You can begin testing for yourself that we truly are connected to everything. I had put forth so much energy into the figure 8 and I had the focus and thoughts of others as well which made drawing it back to me the lessons that this energy teaches even more powerful. There is always a caution to be humble and responsible when tapping into this power, be careful about what you put into your circle. I see now that women who were termed witches, (the ones who followed nature's intended path, without ego's) learned how to work with this energy and had a code that is still used amongst the Wicca tradition today. "Do what you will, with harm to none."

Because of this discovery I now state my intention by first saying thank you. I totally trust what I want will come to me. Then I wait with excitement and anticipation. This excitement is what helps us be in the state that all great mystics have told us, be like a child. The childlike state is when you ask for you desire and then you detach into the mindset of wonder. I wonder how the Universe will bring me my desire. The Goddess is the greatest creatrix and loves to show off if we let her. I remember a time I used to ask the angels to show off to me and it worked and was quite fun receiving the results. Traditionally the end of an intention, invocation or statement was with the words, So Mote it be, or So be it, meaning end of transmition, or you are signing out with the divine forces. For a more modern sense of this word we can look to the Star Trek series with Captain Jon-Luke Picard. At the end of many shows he would use the phrase, "Make it so". This is a great line to use at the end of your intention; then he would sometimes add the word "engage", or in other words... Begin now.

Intentions are a way of speeding up your goal; you are more strongly, focused. Meaning you would be more actively engaged. When you really desire something you spend more hours thinking about it, obsessing if you will. The more you want something the more energy you put behind it. It is this focused energy that attracts what you desire in quicker ways. All doubts have been released and there is only positive expectancy that you will have your intention or something even better. You would not only say your affirmations, you would write them down over and over, like lines on a chalk board. Only this isn't a punishment once handed out in school, it is a repetition for your powerful mind to speed things up.

Your visualizations are more detailed, you move on to the next step which is imagery; which engages all your senses and then you gain more clarity by dwelling on what you want.

Something else to note is that other people have their own agendas or intentions for us. Their intentions may be so strong they seem to dominate over ours, especially when we are first walking the path of becoming. To change the world through a game of golf may seem a bit far fetched, but through a game we learn the lessons of life. I found a wonderful poem that may help your intentions and spirit stay strong and true if you are swayed by people for any number of reasons.

Conflict Resolutions for Life:

People are unreasonable, illogical and self-centered. Love them anyway.
If you do good, people may accuse you of selfish motives. Do good anyway.
If you are successful, you may win false friends and true enemies. Succeed anyway.
The good you do today may be forgotten tomorrow. Do good anyway.
Honesty and transparency make you vulnerable. Be honest and transparent anyway.
What you spend years building may be destroyed overnight. Build anyway.
People who really want help may attack you if you help them. Help them anyway.
Give the world the best you have and you may get hurt. Give the world your best anyway.
The world is full of conflict, choose peace of mind anyway.

- Anonymous

Part 5
Direction Center - Element Ether

Goddess of the Void –
Tara a Tibetan Goddess

Represents the Soul
Ceremony- Daily

Yoga Poses-Mountain pg 159, Standing Yoga Mudra -pg.200

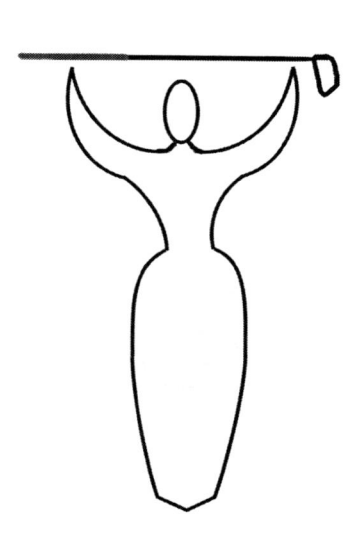

Chapter 9

Tara – Ether Goddess Centering and The Zone

Myth- Tara is the best-known feminine deity of Buddhism. She is said to have taken a vow to help and save others while always remaining in female form.

Poem to Tara
*I sit with my attention focused on my breath
breathing in and out
inhaling and exhaling
taking in and letting go
the dance of creation
the dance of the universe
the dance of life
I sit in stillness
in focused awareness
breathing in and out
as the ocean that is life
churns and pulses around me
as oceans of incarnations
swirl and twirl through me beside me
all around me
My eyes see all
know all
and watch
As I breathe
Sill. Focused. Aware. Centered.*

Lesson of the Goddess
Tara is here to remind you to center. It is time to nourish wholeness by going within and strengthening your center by focusing your awareness. Let the turmoil of life go on without you. It is hard to hear your own voice in the midst of the frenzy of life. Go into the quiet, go into the calm. When you return you will be stronger and more capable of dancing with what life has to offer.
http://www.angelfire.com/va/goddesses/tara/html

Goddess Tara representing the Front Nine

Hole 9 - Centering

It is here we come to our inner space of our heart centre, traditionally after the 9th or 18th hole golfers have completed the course, the circle and return to the clubhouse. Let us view the clubhouse as our inner house. The space that holds our inner core, we have left it to go on a journey around the course and then we come back inside. Spiraling our energy out while playing and then spiraling the energy back into ourselves to our center when we finish. Over time we learn how to Center ourselves in that place of quiet, to be able to spiral back into our center whenever we want and while doing anything. As we prepare to go back to the clubhouse we return to our heart and see what is going on inside us.

When we come forth from a sacred heart and bring that into our playing then we are coming from a grateful heart. We know that when we live and play in sacredness it doesn't mean we are above or below anyone. It means we are being respectful to all beings because they all deserve respect all humans, the earth, the animals, etc. and we come back to community represented by the clubhouse. When we come back with a clean heart we are delicate with our words. We think before we speak, one good practice to remember is if you are going to say something negative bite your tongue, literally. If you feel pain then another person will feel the pain. This way we develop a warrioress attitude to be able to stay awake or else the heart stays asleep. I watched a video years ago and wrote this part down for my classes and I feel you the reader will also benefit from these words.

"The athlete who is in championship form has a quiet place in him/herself, it is out of that place where the action comes from. If you are coming from the chatter in your head or in the controlling state, you are not performing properly. There is a center out of which you act. The center has to be found, otherwise tension comes. Pressure by outside influences - desire, fear, social structures - all impede your performance. If you are coming from your true self, your center, you stay peaceful."
– Joseph Campell, video tape *Myths and Archetypes.*

Come, Be Golfing Goddesses!

The first principle I teach in of all my yoga classes is to bring the students to the present moment. They usually come in to yoga class with their heads full of events from the day. I guide them through a letting go with relaxation/centering to rid them of the stresses, worries, and to help them release conversations in their head about the day's events. Through this consistent practice they begin to develop the experiences of what being in the moment feels like and when the mind wanders off they can recognize the old habit easier and come back to what's happening in the moment. This then becomes a time-out for the maxed out mind and a reacquaintance each time to the connection to the body's language and wisdom. The principle of being in the moment is comparable to having a beginners mind.

We are ahead of the game if we are a beginner because we are not thinking about past yoga experiences and comparing them, in short we don't have to get out of our own way. By that I mean quieting the mind of expectations, or doubts that hinder our performance. This is not only true in yoga, but in golf or any area that we are trying something for the first time. Beginners Luck is not really luck at all; it is being open and accepting.

It is because the energy you put forth is unencumbered, more pure if you will, so events happen effortlessly. Letting go of the past and the future and thinking only of this day, this moment as a new experience is so freeing. We can and will be able to transfer this principle to the game of golf. Others may begin to call you lucky, but you will have a deeper knowing that it is not pure chance that is improving your game.

"I always listen to Margarit's CD on my way to the golf course, and, instead of shaking out of my shoes on the first tee in a competition or match, I am now very calm. All my opponents hate me because they have never seen me hit the ball so well! And the finger relaxation with the re-lax breathing helps tremendously throughout the whole round."
- Charlie Baker (YFG- Level 1)

Similarly most golfers I know arrive at the golf course coming from a state of mental busyness. It does take practice to still the chatterbox, even when we focus on the moment; all kinds of conversations go on and on. You may recognize it as sounding something like this, "Well if I shoot in the low 90's today I will have my lowest score this year. Then I can tell John. He will definitely want to come golfing with me next time. I wonder why so many people are taking a cart today? It's a beautiful day to walk. I'm glad my foursome likes to walk. I hope the group in front of us aren't slow players. I hate it when the group behind us can't see that it's us who has to wait as well and try to hurry us up, etc, etc, etc."

The challenge is to learn to be the observer and become aware when the thoughts ramble. It's okay to watch them as long as we don't invest any emotion behind them. Once again, centering helps ground us to our bodies and to the moment to quiet the inner dialogue. The purpose is to slow down and to detach from distractions, either internal or external. We can also look at centering as the thought process of understanding how every aspect of the game contributes to the overall development and growth as an athlete. It is a kind of concentration that is all encompassing. Shirley Spork, who was on the LPGA in the 1950's and pioneer of the LPGA teaching division, wrote: *"Those who are winning are attuned to everything, the wind, the grass, the sounds, everything. It isn't about blocking out, it's about taking in. It's being so fully aware of the moment that you're protected by it."*

This helps to point out there's nothing unusual or mystical about meditation or being mindful. All it involves is paying attention to your experience moment to moment. This leads to new ways of seeing and being in your life because the present moment, whenever it is recognized and honored, reveals a very special and indeed magical power, it is the only time any of us ever has. The present moment is the only time we have to truly know anything. When we can release two victim phrases from our head "What if" and "If only" we will be able to live more in the present moment. Some golfers never take responsibility for the moment they rely on 'what if' and 'If only,' "*If only* I was a member at a golf club I would improve immensely.", "*What if* I started the game years ago - I would be further along by now." you get the point! On and on the excuses can go, driving us crazy and setting up internal tension. Relax. Remember everything is always cyclical, some days you are on top of your game and some days you're not. Just as the pros have some years they are on top and some years they are not.

Use this next exercise every time you play golf and you will be a calm and composed golfer playing from your true self.

On the golf course we want to use the following exercise. It is a tool that my students use with great results any time golf throws challenges at them. The feedback is mainly when golfers are in tournaments they appreciate the following exercise the most. Whenever they need to recover quickly from a setback, or if they are focused on other people's scores or on the end result, it brings them back to a calm, centered self anytime.

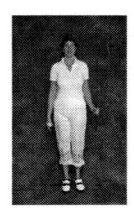

Mountain Pose- Mountain is the foundation for all yoga standing poses.

Mountain – this first exercise will give you a clue about how grounded or ungrounded you are.

1. Begin by standing with feet hip distance apart
2. First raise up the big toes only (notice as you concentrate to do this you hold your breath. KEEP BREATHING throughout this exercise and every other in this book. When we hold our breath it keeps the body tight and tense - the opposite of what we want. W are stretching out our bodies.
3. Now lower your big toes, leave them planted to the ground and raise up the small toes at once. Breathe
4. Lower them, Now raise up all the toes at once. I bet this is easier to do.
5. Immediately become aware that your body shifted a bit to the front. If you did not, get this sense do the exercise again. This is where we begin with the foundation, with the weight evenly balanced between the heels and the balls of the feet.
6. Now if you are one of the rare persons that had no problem connecting with your toes, you are pretty grounded. For most, one or the other is easier and some can only do number 4 successfully.
7. Bend the knees slightly and tuck in your pelvis.
8. Imagine a string at the base of the spine and it pulls up all the way to the crown of the head and above a few inches. Imagine a marionette puppet being pulled up straight.

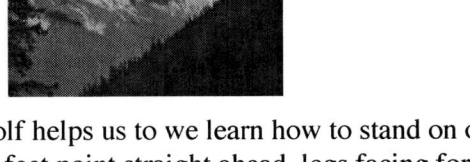

Mountain pose in yoga for golf helps us to we learn how to stand on our own two feet. We are planted, our feet point straight ahead, legs facing forward never leaning on one leg or another.

Being Mindful of the Qualities of a Mountain can bring thoughts such as: majestic, solid, stable, sacred.

Physiological benefits are – builds confidence, stability and endurance.

Physical benefits – develops concentration, co-ordination, balance, poise and strength.

This stance is used to ground and center ourselves. We begin to center ourselves by training our body, mind and emotions with what in yoga is called a mantra and a mudra. A mantra is a word or phrase repeated over and over. The word we are going to use is Relax. When it is combined with the breath it has a very powerful effect at calming the mind and emotions. With the breath in repeat REEEEEEeeeeee- with the out going breath say LLLLLLLLLAAAAAAAAxxxxx. This is all done quietly in your mind not out loud as one can get a fuller inhale and long deeper exhale. Also, whenever possible, the breath will always be in and out through the nostrils.

Then we add the mudra which acts as an anchor It is with practice of relaxed feelings that you will be able to call upon them any time during waking hours. This is especially beneficial to bring you back to a calm state where all decision-making is at the optimal.

Mudra- If you are a right handed golfer you would use your right hand and opposite if you are left handed. Train either with or without a golf ball in your hand. Form a circle with the thumb and pointer finger and the remaining three fingers point straight downwards.

Mudra means seal…… Joining the thumb and pointer finger together is a seal of our human selves joined together with the God Force …

"I played yesterday and a couple of times I was on the tee thinking of a recent shot rather than being focused on the present and I realized what I was doing. I took that opportunity to use the finger relaxation focus and took a moment just to take two deep inhale/exhales and both times the drive was great. I think I may have to add the 2 breath routine to all my tee pre-shot routine".

Thanks, Mike Creed

Anytime emotions are high on the golf course from first tee nerves, to frustration or trying to hurry, this will be invaluable to center yourself. Why? Because whatever words we send to ourselves, our bodies respond to automatically, whether we are paying attention or not. By simply saying relax, the body does.

Let's look at this truth that I use a few times throughout this book, "Your body makes the shot, but it is the mind that controls the body." Too many instructions at once can overload the brain making your swings look sloppy and choppy. It is okay to be a hacker when first learning the game, but think back to the analogy of first learning to drive a standard car. When first learning with the conscious mind the movements are not smooth when driving, Too many instructions all at once. Discovering this type of playing golf, trusting the body, helps us break free of the unconscious message steeped in this sport, that we always need to fix our swing. The messages in learning the game have been unbalanced with the emphasis on left brain, intellectual thinking of the mechanics of the game. Your body does develop muscles memory and can hit the ball well if we can get out of our thinking mind.

Try this simple experiment to show you the best example of how your words command your body.

1. Facing forward take your right arm straight out in front of you and point a finger.
2. Turning to the right as far as you can, when you stop look at what your finger is pointing to and then bring the arm back to the front of the body.
3. Saying out loud the command "go farther"
4. Repeat step two and Lo and Behold the arm goes farther.
5. Let's do the other side (because yoga is all about balance - whatever you do on one side you do on the other).

If you really want to have fun, repeat step one and two and then for
Step 3, command your arm to "Go as far as you can"; now turn the body. Amazing how it can still go a bit further.

NOW just think, you didn't have to give any instructions mentally to your body to turn further, it just naturally knew how to turn more. For example the knees bent all on their own to assist the turn. Are you starting to get the point, Trust your body!

This exercise can even be used with fun at the driving range. Hit a ball and then say to the next one, "Go further." My command over the last few years when I am playing is to mentally tell the ball "Go as straight and as far as you can". It works beautifully. Try it out, little things like this help you play more. Playing while playing the game brings more spontaneity and fun to our games, it helps break us free from mundane playing.

Again the importance of keeping things simple is crucial. Give the command with the conscious brain, so whatever word we chose the sub-conscious says Yes to and follows the command. If we are saying the word Re-laxxx the body will begin to soften and let go effortlessly because at a sub-conscious level it instinctively knows how to relax.

Goddess Tara representing the Back Nine

Hole 18 - The Zone

"An ounce of Perception equals a ton of Education" –The Void

We look to Eastern Philosophy to help describe the mystery of the Zone.

When we think of the void usually we visualize blackness and the dark, the unknown which most of us do not embrace. Black was once honored as a sacred color of the Goddess. Black is the maternal color, it is the womb out of which the new is born. Black is the color of creation. This information, as well as all Goddess knowledge, is still buried deep in our bones, the memories from our ancestors.

The zone is becoming easier to describe now that the East and West are becoming more integrated. The zone is generally described as elusive and mysterious, which are feminine traits. I have come to learn that Golf is best played with a more Yin approach. To play in the mystery/The Zone is to be in the feminine. To be happy in golf you will find more enjoyment by playing in the Yin energy, to be Yielding and Humble. Instead of using words like elusive to describe the zone, I think a more fitting word would be esoteric-which translates to, 'That which is hidden.' The best description I have heard for the meaning of esoteric is the example of an iceberg. When you see an iceberg from shore you are only looking at 10% of it, 90% of it is hidden underwater.

Just like when we see a person's head we see 10% of it, the outside. The real important stuff is the 90% on the inside. Let us get somewhat acquainted with the inside. To help us with this understanding let's look at the three different states of our mind, the conscious mind, the sub-conscious mind and the super-conscious mind.

The Conscious Mind perceives, reasons, judges, rejects; it has a conscious communication with the body through the five senses.

The Sub-Conscious Mind controls the involuntary processes of the operation of the body: digestion, beating of the heart, blood circulation, it builds, sustains and repairs it. It is a storehouse for memory, habit and instinct. It could be considered the follower of the conscious mind. A very powerful one at that, and it is very agreeable to the thoughts, words and images the conscious mind and super conscious mind feed it, whether they are for our best interest or not. To reinstate what was said earlier in this book, the sub-conscious doesn't judge, it just agrees to follow whatever direction it is given.

The Super-Conscious Mind is more connected to our hearts and to our souls; it is associated with the higher inspiring ideas, creativity, and imagination. When we meditate on the point between the eyebrows we are helping to open to our super-consciousness, the intuitive side of ourselves. When inspiration dawns, that first thought is from Spirit, the second and third thoughts are the doubts coming from the conscious mind. When we doubt, we lose out. But it is only through mistakes that we see the truth of this and then we can correct our actions to follow our Spirit the next time it prompts us.

I have been in the zone a few times while golfing but the time that really stuck with me, when I could actually see the line for my putts and I willed the ball into the hole was playing in a charity tournament. The other three women were better golfers so I practiced my internal golf for a few days prior to the tournament. With this practice and then the added sound of a farmers equipment going that echoed throughout the golf course all day was like a steady drum beat helped to shift me into a more grounded and peaceful state.

So that is my story on the zone probably different then any you have heard. But one important point that is common for all golfers is it is hard to get in the zone with a bad attitude. I mentioned this quote before and it is worth repeating, Payne Stewart said, "A bad attitude is worse than a bad swing."

Legend of Bagger Vance – The Movie – depicts how when Bobby was in the field (Zone) he was swinging his club and "searching". Bagger tells Junah, "He is searching for that perfect swing, and It is out there. He has many to choose from - flops and hooks, duffers and slices and then good ones to great ones. The perfect one wants him just as much as he wants it. It is only through being calm and composed can one bring it into physical form."

What I was told over and over again, while taking my yoga teacher training, which I would like to impart to you in my own words; "the Goddess already sees you as perfect you are her child and she loves you and accepts you for who you are right here and right now. Can you? You have gifts inside of you, you have infinite beauty and infinite power. Her goal for you is the same as yours, which is to be happy. To live your highest vision, to become the best you, you have many experiences in the ether, which ones are you going to draw down into your life?

The problem seems to stem from our gift of free will this wouldn't be a problem if we weren't so conditioned by our cultures. It boils down to only you can make the decision to be happy. It all begins inside of you, but because we are bombarded by fear because of years of control we need to break out of this mold first, so we can choose from inside of us what we truly deserve.

When fear and its many faces seem overwhelming you can use a meditation that channeled through for me when I was going through a particular rough patch. At the time I was conditioned to think of looking outside of me to find a way to feel better, to be happy. Buy, Buy, Buy is what I had been shown was the path to happiness. But on this day my conscious mind and my super conscious mind had a conversation on their own and I was just observing. My conscious mind listed all of the ways I could feel better. I thought, "I'll go out and buy a new outfit;" my super conscious mind responded, "No, I have enough clothes, I went through thoughts of buying other things, each time some part of me said No, that will only make me happy for a short time." I then went on to food and drink each time, a big No. Fine I thought I will call and vent to a friend. One this day not one person was home. (Since that time, I have noticed other times I have gone through crises and called for support and no one is home. I realize that the Goddess wants me to tune in and go directly to the source for comfort instead of my friends at these times)

I was frustrated so I closed my eyes and took a few deep breaths and the next thing I knew I was going through a meditation, or a story in my head. I pass this on to you to use anytime there are fearful situations confronting you regarding your personal life, business life or play time.

Try it at home first with your eyes closed and when you have the concept down you can use it anytime you need to overcome fear. I did make a recording of it which you can download as an mp3 and will probably find more effective at first because it has more detail but this is still an effective means of training may your imagination.

We all visualize in our mind by seeing pictures. If I was to say, "Picture a dog", you would see a dog, not the word. Otherwise we have to consciously want to see words, and in this visualization we do.

Begin by seeing yourself at a chalkboard and now write out the word Fear.

FEAR in big letters. Now see yourself erase that and write the word courage, EVEN BIGGER, COURAGE and Bolder if you like.
Now write the word fear once more but smaller this time, fear

Erase it and replace it with the word POWER. Use a different color chalk for this word, what color would you use?

Finally write fear so small it just takes a flip of the wrist to erase it- fear

Next, imagine you can write the word LOVE the length of your body.

The L as long as you are, the O the width of you, and the V and E the length of you.

Now with your powerful imagination see the color of Love.

See it go out and surround what you are fearful of at this time so it can come back to you bringing the highest energy of healing for yourself and what you fear.

Feel alive with courage, power and love and know that everything is working for the highest good.

Do not let fear stop you from enjoying all the beauty, love, and abundance the wonderful planet has to offer.

A truth about fear is that it leaves as soon as we face it. One good way of thinking of fear is:

FALSE
EVIDENCE
APPEARING
REAL
- Zig Zigler

This has helped me enormously when I have been fearful. Remember if you are having a difficult time and no one is around to talk to and comfort you. There is still the Goddess and she may want you to tune in and meditate or talk to her." I heard the translation for meditate is wisdom, and we are told that all our answers are inside ourselves. It only takes us to be still long enough to gain the insights. A gift like this meditation proves to me how much the Goddess loves us, the evidence becomes more real the more we pay attention. The exciting thing about living in our times is that now the new science Quantum Physics is supporting the ancient Spiritual teachings. The Spiritual teachings tell us, begin to observe yourself as happy and that observation will expand and become your reality. Begin to observe how much you are loved and supported by the Goddess and it will become your reality.

The world shows us our thoughts. The greatest gift we have is the power to change our minds. We don't have to search for more, we are enough, nothing outside can make you perfect, You already are. Become conscious of your true self, the perfect you, is already there, it's just hidden like the iceberg. Become conscious of the zone, it is already there just waiting to be called forth.

I think why I like the Movie What the Bleep do we know over The Secret is it is a more gentle in its informative approach. This description of the New Science of Quantum Physics which I copied here from the movie might help you to grasp the esoteric language more deeply.

"We are conditioned to believe that our world outside of ourselves is independent of our experiences. It is not. Quantum physicists have been so clear about it. Einstein himself, the co-discoverer of Quantum Physics, said, "atoms are not things, they are only tendencies." So instead of things, we have to think of possibilities.'

Another pair of women I recognize the "Goddess of Golf" working through is Pia Nilson and Lynn Marriot, they have created a program called 'Vision 54' and they teach golfers to believe in all possibilities. Golf is one way back to the heart, back to Spirit and living in rapture. How, by teaching us to allow all our senses to guide us, even the sixth sense. If you forget this remember results are always changing from hole to hole, from shot to shot. The mountain pose can help you be like an esoteric iceberg that keeps you cool and collective. You will understand in a whole new way the phrase "Grace under pressure." Concentrate at the task at hand and then let it go, keep good thoughts in your head between shots.

Keep good thoughts in your head between games. And one day you will notice golfers will start to call you lucky because you make everything look easy and effortless. But you will know that the saying, "Only the unenlightened use the word lucky". Luck is preparation, meeting opportunity. Following these steps, whether in golf, life or business, you are on your way to living from your highest potential. Rumi, a Sufi poet stated, "Inside every human being are Gods and Goddesses in embryo and there is only one desire, they want to be born." Your inner Gods and Goddesses can lift you from an ordinary experience into a magical game, Raise your vibration by being in nature and this will transfer to living in a magical world in every area of your life.

Now that we have understood the steps to describe the zone how do we go into it. I will ask you to watch the movie The Legend of Bagger Vance for one clue. When Bagger asks if Junah is ready to see the field, this is your cue to listen carefully and you will understand that the field means being in the zone. *Bagger tells Junah, "I can't bring you to it I can only point the way. It is not about thinking your way to it, intellectualizing your way to it. It is about focusing and grounding to your center it is about feeling with your hands not your head."*

One practice you might begin which I haven't tried myself as I just got the insight is to release language. Be the witness, feel each experience and don't name it. When you make a beautiful drive do not name it, do not put words to it just experience it, feel it, and savor it. In Deepka Chopra's version of the Bhagvad Gita he tells us that we have a tape loop going around and around in our heads of pure conditioning and it is playing back to us 24,000 words a day. How do we break away from the tape loop?

Awareness of it, throughout the book you have been giving tools of how words, our language, can heal or destroy. This brings us back to the beginning of this book. When I mentioned that I had a vision to help people to control their thoughts because time was speeding up and what we focus on will happen quicker then ever before. In the last eight years I have witnessed the truth of this Vision. Maybe if we drop naming our things and experiences we will see them with fresh new eyes. In the next few years it will be important to make a discipline of seeing the glass half full, there will be many distractions. We have the capabilities to be one human family in which we will all live up to our truest selves.

Think of all the Masters who have come before us, all had to go through temptations before the breakthrough to true Mastery. Living a Spiritual warrioress path takes courage and discipline to overcome the different degrees of fear that arises as we go around and around through the cycles, the important step is to keep letting go of one way of becoming to the go to the next layer of becoming. Mini deaths and rebirths over and over, a person should never stay stuck on any level, there is no real goal, just the adventure. Raja yoga and Patanjali warn against staying stuck on the path. One must remain Humble and not want to aim with the ego, which hates change.

The ego can want to achieve to the level of being a Magician and materialize objects out of thin air. But I ask you, where is the higher love on that path? No, I have witnessed we are not meant to stay only on one path, that reflects our thinking mode, in a straight line. To walk the path of the Masters is to keep walking, and following behind the lead of Nature. I asked you at the beginning of the book to begin your search as seeing golf as a spiritual path, and a path to the heart, a hero's path. I have learned through living and writing this book, that as I keep trusting nature to point the way towards my purpose in life the searching stopped, and I became one with the questions and answers. When most people are beginning the search into "Who am I?" and "Why am I here?" The popular answer from books and teachers is, "A journey begins with one step." And it is up to each individual to make the step on their own, the exciting part is when they do, they can find support everywhere. My experience has taught me a second part to the popular saying,

"While on the journey, Never stop walking and the search will reveal itself over and over again."

This Golf Goddess energy has been a wonderful guide and has helped me grow into my own Goddess self through this creative journey of bringing her into being through the art of writing. And I have been in the zone while writing many times a powerful story for me that I would like to share happened when I arrived back in B.C. after visiting my family in Ontario 2007 at Christmas Time. Even though I have faithfully followed my inner Goddess promptings, many times I have not wanted to. Now I am not saying I did not want to come to B.C., I did, but I felt I was pushed into it before I was ready to let go of my kids. I have always felt a small hole in my heart where some guilt and sadness for leaving my children perks its head up. I could not fully be free to enjoy myself completely on this adventure. I believe the Goddess has seen into my heart and given me some Christmas magic to help heal me just a little bit more.

When my partner and I went back to Ontario for Christmas in 2007 I thought this book was completed. But I see now the Goddess just gave me some time off, because when parts of this book want to get written, like this last part I am adding, I get no rest until I follow through. So, in saying, I did not have thoughts about the book at all, I had the freedom to be fully in the moments with my wonderful children. I wish I had the gift of a poet to properly describe the emotion of being with my children again, how far the depth of the sorrow is when I am not with them, especially on key dates like birthdays, but then it all goes away and profound deepness of joy surrounds us when they are in my arms again. I truly understand how pain and joy have become one.

Leaving my children was much harder then going through the process of my parent's quick death. And all of it took place within a couple of years of each other. Once again I tell you this move has been the hardest path to follow. At the same time though I have loved living in B.C. it is the best province for a nature lover, and I know the beauty has been a big inspiration for this book. Now that I am back in this home, my heart is not so heavy, I know my children are happy and settled in their own lives, yes, they miss me, but they do not really need me. The gift of comfort and blessings the Goddess has bestowed on me, is by showing me very clearly, I am right where I need to be, even though I knew I was, I still needed these meaningful coincidences to help me live with more enthusiasm about my path.

And the circle goes round and round…..At the beginning of this book I had mentioned what happened to me after being at a Wayne Dyer workshop and now this book ends with listening to a Wayne Dyer talk New Years Day. I started off the New Year saying "2008 is going to be Great!" and my notice of this affirmation came immediately. I am so grateful Wayne supports Public Television because I wouldn't have seen him otherwise. We just arrived from the airport and my partner put on the t.v. then, fell asleep. I had control of the remote and shows I wanted to watch, if any, but the box worked for me that day. As soon as I saw Wayne Dyer's name I was very excited. He is a great inspiration for me because he walks the path of the heart and I view him like an older brother who helps point the way. The theme for the show was inspiration, it was so appropriate on many levels.

Wayne then began to share an incredible story, he said he was completing the book on Inspiration and that he wanted it to have 18 chapters because he believes 18 is a very significant number. The number 8 is a symbol for infinity and he defines it by viewing when you put a one in front of the 8 then you are 'being at one with the infinite.' He told how the Bagavad Gita has 18 chapters and how a Golf Course has 18 holes. My ears perked as you can imagine. What was even more significant was that he finished the book on his birthday May 10th, which is my birthday! Wow, but it gets even deeper for me. Wayne then goes on to describe that the chapter he just wrote about was on a Monarch Butterfly. My mother loved butterflies she was a great quilter and had put many butterflies in her wall hangings. All her friends always gave her butterflies as gifts.

Wayne is describing his friend Jack who loved butterflies and how his friend had passed away. Then he called his editor and said the book was completed and went out for a walk along the beach. The story from here is quite long but the amazing part for Wayne was a butterfly flew on his finger and stayed with him for hours. He was able to have some pictures taken with the butterfly and it is on the front cover of his book named Inspiration. He believed it was his friend Jack, I was moved by this but I only saw it as a symbol for the New Year as butterflies are viewed as transformation. From being a caterpillar, going through the transformation in the cocoon state to finally emerging with wings to fly. It seemed to be what has happened with the writing of my book and now I was ready to fly.

But that is not all the message meant for me. The next segment Wayne was sharing about where his inspiration came from and one of the people was his Mother. She was in the audience and she reminded me of my mother because of her red hair. Then it dawned on me I was receiving a message from my mother. A couple of days earlier Sylvia Brown was on T.V. answering peoples questions and she said our loved ones always come visit around holidays and special occasions. It made sense that I mom would get a message to me that she was thinking of me with love, because at the airport earlier that morning when saying goodbye to my daughter it was such a raw feeling of pain for both of us.

Although unlike the last goodbye when moving out here, this time I really went into the feeling and didn't push it away. I allowed the tears to move through me and it was very healing. I had said goodbye to my son the day before but he instructs me that I am not allowed to cry in front of him because it upsets him. I will have to let him know next time that it is important to feel all the feelings when they are happening instead of stuffing them.

So of course while watching and sending love to my parents I had another good cry, knowing that they are still with me, but in a different way now but still very much a part of our lives. The final coincidence that happened that day which gave me the assurance that I am living where I am suppose to be at the moment to bring forth this book. The movie –' The Legend of Bagger Vance' came on immediately after.

Now I have watched this many times but that day many of the teachings throughout the movie had more meaning for me. I think in part because of being shifted to a higher place by first watching Wayne Dyer and because I had just been writing about the movie in this last chapter. And if you recall Wayne said the Bagavad Gita has 18 chapters, the golf course has 18 holes and this last theme is number 18 in this book. Wow!

Now at the very last moment of bringing this book to delivery, I received it back from the publishers to sign off that it was ready to go live. My daughter went into early Labor and had a baby girl, my granddaughter, Kaitlyn Mary was born nine days early (just in time to be added to this last editing) she arrived November 18, 2008.

With her early arrival I had another insight by adding the two numbers - one plus eight together like the spiritual science of numerology does. It equals nine, one aspect of the number nine represents completion. The circle comes back to completion, just like on the golf courses. I feel the year 2009 will be a year of many completions, already I am seeing pieces of the puzzle come to completion and my life's journey making sense where it never has before.

As I have mentioned the children are already coming onto this planet awake and aware of their life's mission.

Before I share a future vision for Golfing Goddesses and humanity I need to share a story of my Granddaughter and how she was connected to the web before even arriving. Although she came to me in dreams and a future vision, I also felt love from her the week before she came because I have become even more highly sensitive. This is not so for my daughter who did receive a message from her unborn child back in September. She went to Sears to register for her baby shower and was waiting in line. A mother and her daughter (about four years of age) were in front of her and when they were leaving the little girl turned to my daughter and said "Kate says Hi." The mother said, "Who is Kate," and her daughter replied, "it doesn't matter." And they walked away, leaving my daughter as she explained, 'creeped out'. If my daughter was awake (aware) and trusting she would have registered for a baby girl. However, I am confident between me, her mother and now her daughter she will become much more awake! After meeting my granddaughter I see she is already a Goddess, she was born one like we all were. I dream that one day we will be able to connect properly to the new children and to our inner child. To connect with on a real level and to help midwife what the children are passionate about, even if we do not understand it. Those passions are the link to their life purpose and could be a doorway that may lead to the paradise and simpler times we all crave.

I leave you now with four words for our future;
"it's all about connecting."

Connecting to – Nature and all its kingdoms, to the seasons, to Mother Earth and Father Sky, to the spirit within all things, to play, to the inner male and female, to the outer male and female, to girlfriends, to children, to Grandparents, to the ancestors, to Divinity, to the intangible, to the breath, to the virtues, to peace, to the heart and unconditional love, to a global community, to the sweet spot, to golf courses.

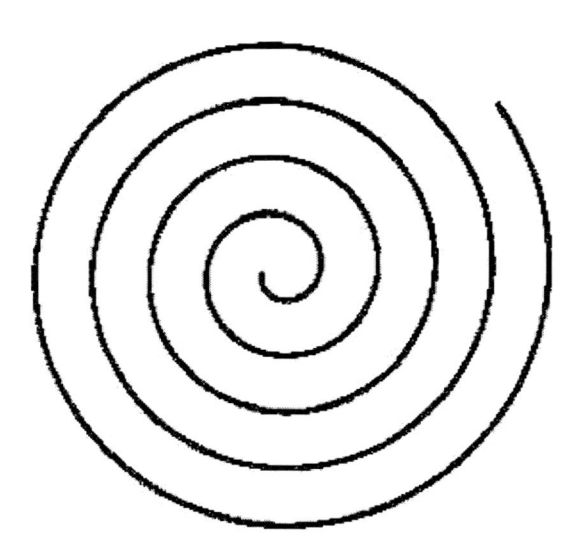

Come, Be Golfing Goddesses!

Sacred Golf Journeys
A New Dawn- The Future Is Golden

"The world will be saved by the Western woman."
—H.H., The Dalai Lama

I believe I understand this quote by the Dalai Lama to mean the western woman can help save the world since we have the financial means to do so, we are gaining more spiritual insight so we desire to heal ourselves along with the earth, and there is more freedom in our lives to be of greater service.

Personally I would change it to the 'western women' since we will be able to shift quicker as we come together to help the world through our unity. I have been able to reflect about my book being a birthing process from my daughter's pregnancy and the delivery for this book has been similar to having a baby. There have been the labor pains and the pushing involved at the end, I even had to go to my new friend Pamela Brand's home for a few days so I could be with a woman to help midwife the last stages of this books delivery, much to the confusion and bewilderment of my partner. My whole being pressured me to leave my home and my heart was a bit heavy until the Goddess sent me some confirming signs that this is what she required of me. I will share one sign that came in the form of an email. The unfortunate thing with email messages that get passed around is you don't always know the original source. So I take the risk to add it now and to share how very grateful I am to the person who wrote it. I share it especially for all the loving supportive women who have come in and out of my life, who have always been there for me, and who I believe always will be!

Email-
Time passes. Life happens. Distance separates. Children grow up.
Jobs come and go. Love waxes and wanes.
Men don't do what they're supposed to do.
Hearts break. Parents die. Colleagues forget favors. Careers end.
BUT.........
Sisters are there, no matter how much time and how
many miles are between you.
A girl friend is never farther away than needing her can reach.
When you have to walk that lonesome valley and you

*have to walk it by yourself, the women in your life
will be on the valley's rim, cheering you on,
praying for you, pulling for you, intervening on
your behalf, and waiting with open arms at the valley's end.*

*Sometimes, they will even break the rules and walk
beside you...Or come in and carry you out.
Girlfriends, daughters, granddaughters,
daughters-in-law, sisters, sisters-in-law, Mothers,
Grandmothers, aunties, nieces, cousins, and extended family, all
bless our life!
The world wouldn't be the same without women, and
neither would I. When we began this adventure called
womanhood, we had no idea of the incredible joys or
sorrows that lay ahead. Nor did we know how much we
would need each other.
Every day, we need each other still.*

Questing to Sacred Sites
As incredible as it sounds the game of golf can set us on the path to delivering a New Earth in an easy and joyful way. How will this be accomplished? By women connecting together and questing or going on a pilgrimage to the sacred birth places of the Goddesses.

I know I am blessed into usefulness by being a connector, or a bridge, to help women live magical lifestyles as they connect back to the land in a sacred way.

In Jean Shinoda Bolen's book "Crossing to Avalon" she explains it this way:

"The search is a part of the quickening. By being a pilgrim on this Goddess Quest is to go to sacred places to quicken the divinity within to experience a spiritual awakening, or receive a blessing or become healed. The seeker embarks on a journey with a receptive soul and hopes to find divinity there."

Yes! Many have found and are living in divinity. As luck would have it, there are golf courses now all over the world connecting golfers as one community. I realize not only will it be great fun to travel for a week with my sisters but I feel compelled to do it to help save the planet. This desire began from me finally understanding the meaning of words 'the microcosm' and 'the macrocosm' this is from seeing it being played out in the western world. Over the past four decades many people have taken their own inner pilgrimages going through the dark night of the soul before reaching the dawn, this is the microcosm, the individual. Many of these people, including myself, have turned around to give a helping hand to help others with their path. Some of the metaphysical understanding came from the fear of the prophecy that foretold the world would end in 2000. Energetically the world did end we have shifted and are now about to shift again in 2012. Since the beginning of 2000 many of the individuals have come more together in groups to raise the energy to help the earth and to bring humanity's energy back towards a more loving and generous nature. At this time we are living collectively as a whole, it is the dark night of the soul for the world, this is the macrocosm, and we will come into the dawn of a spiritual rebirth as a whole. There is a story you may want to research called "The hundredth monkey syndrome" which helps shed light on the phenomenon of enough people doing something the rest will be lifted to the same. The something in our case is to add to the quantum leap of the new world as we quest to sacred sites. In this way we are helping add our energy to the raising of the worlds vibrations towards oneness along with the many other individuals and groups working towards the same goal. Imagine with me if you will;

Journeying to the parts of the world that the nine Goddesses in this book originated from, as Golfing Goddesses we will play in a sacred way on and off the golf courses. We will visit Pele's home in Hawaii and swim with the dolphins and their unconditional love, pure Joy and play. Dolphins are some of the best teachers in the world to teach us the feeling of joy and to understand the sacredness of play!

Another quest will deliver us to Egypt to honor Isis, then on Greece to visit the temples of Artemis, and on and on we will travel spreading our light, love and joyfulness.

A Goddess Garden

The opening of buds signals the beginning of a new season. The Great Goddess is again blooming around the world. Look for her in flowers, laughter, children, elders, the people you meet today, and yourself, look and you will find her. Her buds are green, but her flowers blossom into all the colors of the world.

May we bloom, each in our own way
 Revealing the beauty within
May our ancient roots give us healing strength
Nurturing our best selves.
May we celebrate diversity, respect each person we meet
Understand that we are one family.
May each of us always remember...

*We are united in hope and divided in fear
Put away fear and celebrate our human family.
Like the flowers of the garden, we flourish when we have sunshine, clean water, clean air, room for our roots to grow and many diverse neighbors. Each one adding something unique and special to our experience and environment* -Abby Willowroot
www.spiralgoddesses.com

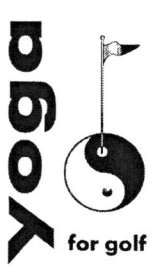

Hatha Yoga- Golf is an asymmetrical game for the body and Hatha yoga's first rule is; what you do on one side of the body you need do on the other. Balance is the key, it helps to prevent injury and to keep the body supple and strong. Yoga is a wonderful practice for the fitness side of golf and many of the poses can help everyone get stronger and feel better regardless of age. Stretching is the key to removing tension and releasing energy. Especially as we age, the gentle body manipulation of yoga is crucial. If older golfers don't stretch you can guarantee their swing will shorten every year and they will lose yardage. Stretching also improves circulation, decreasing the likelihood of degenerative diseases.

Anxiety and tension are feelings that all golfers experience on the golf course, sometimes the problems arise when these inner tensions become an overriding factor in our lives and in our game. The Yoga for Golf stretches help ease muscular tension- this in turn has a calming effect on the mind and body.

In general yoga stretches move at a slower pace than other forms of fitness, bringing discipline and focus which are two essential components required in golf. These golf specific poses focus on the muscles and tendons used in playing the game of golf. The most important lesson to learn is how to incorporate the breathing into synchronization with the body movements.

Two different breaths to be used with the yoga poses-
Please go back and reacquaint yourself with the instructions of Belly Breathing and the Complete Breathe from the theme Pranayama in Chapter Two.

When both breaths are mastered, I teach them to be used in the different asanas. When you are in an easy pose, breathing from your belly helps to keep you in the moment. This is where we always want to be while doing yoga - awareness in the body, in the moment, not thinking about what to make for dinner, or about your family or work.

The Complete Breath is best for more intense poses. The deeper the stretch, the deeper the breath, is what I tell my students. If there is too much tightness in one area of the body, it manifests as pain. The deeper the breath, the more oxygen is being brought to the body, the more the body can relax and lengthen, and more energy is being circulated. The shorter the breath, or Goddess forbid not breathing at all, the tighter the body is.

Breathing in Postures:

Each Posture is more than a physical and technical position. There is a dynamic flow of energy that is created and moved in each posture. Practice should be done with intent and not in a casual or habitual state. Attending to the flow of the breath and energy in the postures helps bring back attention to each posture. One example of being present to the moment is to think about if you have ever watched a cat stalk a bird. Every muscle, every tendon, every heartbeat is focused on the prey. Have you ever watched a cat stretch after a nap? It is the same attention every muscle, every tendon, every heartbeat is totally involved in the stretch. This is our goal in yoga, this is what the ancient yogic forest dwellers observed by watching animals how they moved and then they mimicked the animals and named the poses after them.

1. Maintain deep, even, diaphragmatic breathing. This regulates the nervous system to mediate the stress response. Thus via the sympathetic nervous system, the overall level of muscle tension throughout the body is reduced making release into each pose easier.

2. Breathe slowly and through the nose. This expands the lung capacity giving better oxygen exchange. This also creates the habit of nasal breathing which is always healthier for the body.

3. Keep the breath flowing smoothly. One is less likely to tense muscles if breathing is constant. Holding the breath usually leads to tension and can also lead to misalignment of the spine

4. Move with the breath. Moving downward into a posture or moving into a posture involving flexion, such as a forward or side bend, it is natural to exhale to release tension. Raising up or extending the spine, as you do when you move into the cobra, can be synchronized with a slow

inhalation. To move slowly, try one or more complete breaths. Energy follows attention.

5. While holding a posture, move your attention throughout the length of the entire body in a sweeping pattern with the flow of the breath.
In a posture, use your exhalations to release any tension you find.
Inhale to fill body with vigor and vitality.

Points to Remember
-Breathe freely as you practice these stretches
- stretch-not strain; do not stretch beyond physical comfort. Your flexibility will improve with persistence and consistency.
- As will all exercis programs, consult with your physician first before beginning this program.
- The yoga poses will begin to teach us how to move away from listening to the chattering mind and begin a relationship to listening to the body. While in the poses we keep our focus on feeling what is happening in the body and the steady rhythm of the breath.

Before doing any of the proceeding yoga poses I would like to introduce you to a routine that can be performed in one minute as a stepping stone to build a daily habit of yoga. It can be used at home as a warm-up before golf or used at the golf courses as your warm-up.

Moon Pose Benefits: Increases the flexibility of the spine. Increases ROM in shoulders. Strengthening and toning of every muscle in the central part of the body, ankles, knees, hips, back, shoulders and neck. Firming and trimming of waistline, hips, abdomen, buttocks and thighs.

When the breath and movements are co-coordinated this sequence can be preformed three times in as little as 60 seconds. It can be very easy to put aside 60 seconds in a day. At the beginning of Doing your Dailies, it helps to think of the qualities of the moon to keep this routine gentle. The moon has no gravity, I ask you to consciously use this thought for the movements so your body can become soft, light and loose each time you do it.

*** Point to remember our bodies are stiffer in the mornings and our minds are more alert in comparison to late afternoon when the body is warmed up from movements throughout the day and the mind is quieter.
If practicing the one-minute sequence in the morning you can add a warm-up

such touching the toes repeatedly in a relaxed, light manner.

Doing the Dailies to get started:
One- Minute Moon Sequence

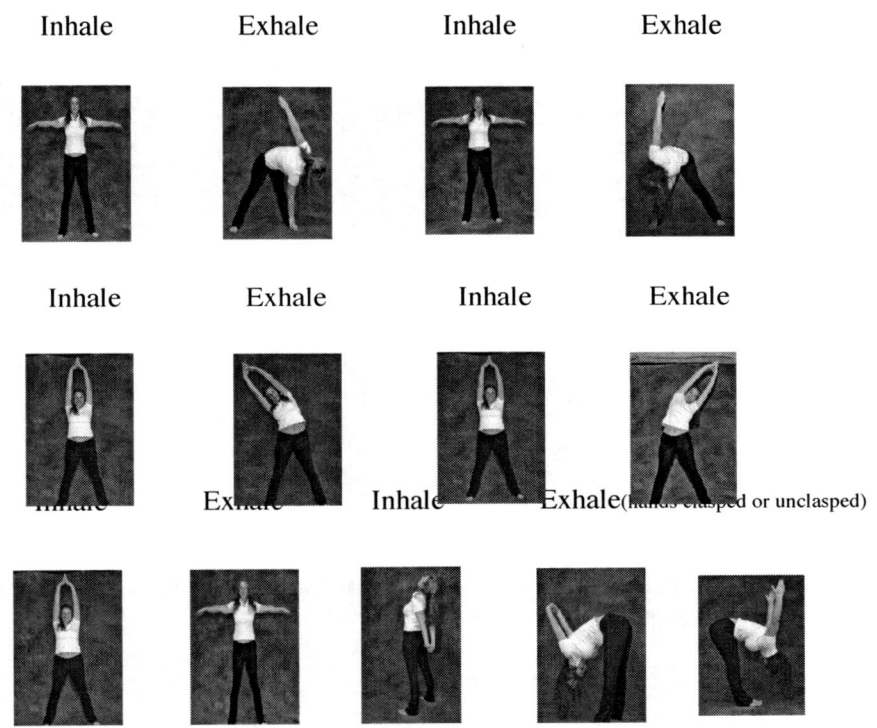

Inhale	Exhale	Inhale	Exhale

Inhale	Exhale	Inhale	Exhale

Exhale   Inhale   Exhale(hands clasped or unclasped)

Doing your Dailies with fun: I have been teaching this movement for a long time to Van Morssion's song 'Moon Dance'. Playing the song and practicing the Moon sequence has become a common bond that I interchange between my regular yoga classes, Yoga for Golf classes, Goddess Yoga classes and now Golfing Goddesses classes. I think this is my favorite yoga movement because it holds memories of all my students combined. Now when ever I hear the song played it always makes me smile and think of teaching yoga and how all my classes have always enjoyed doing this routine to Van's song.

Golfers Warm-ups: warm-ups are a gentle repetitive movement that bring warmth and energy to cold tight muscles helping to prevent injuries.

You may already have your own warm-up routine I've included these few moves that can be performed at the driving range or golf course. An individual could also include some neck stretches or arm circles with or without a golf club. But please remember yoga's first rule; what you do on one side is always practiced on the other.

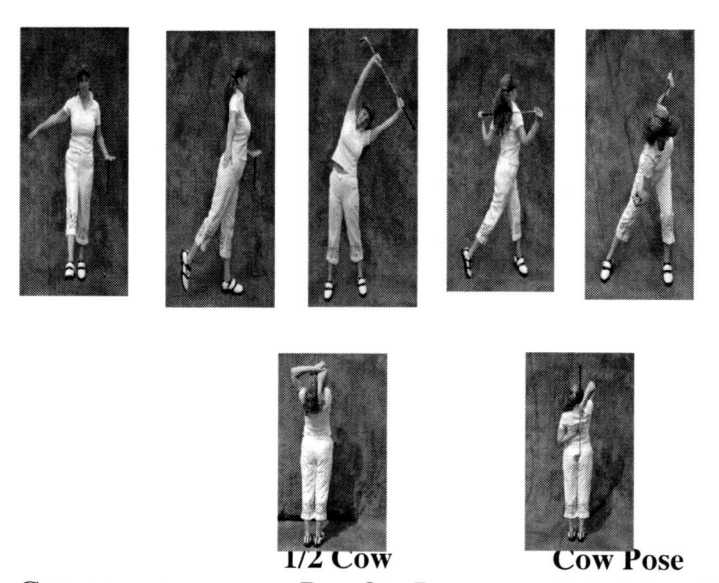

1/2 Cow   Cow Pose
Cow pose as warm-up-Benefits- Loosens and stretches shoulders, rotator cuff, strengthens triceps
Repeat sides

Creating your own Yoga for Golf Routine: just as Mother Earth wants to be back in relationship with her human children, our bodies crave to be back in relationship. Therefore I am starting with the yoga poses in a sequence that can either be done in the order I have arranged them by the elements. Or you allow the wisdom of your body and not this book to direct what you need each time you come to practice.

After a few breaths you state an intention that you are humble before your body and you request the body's wisdom to show you what poses you need for that day. You can even request poses you need for health and healing. With healing ask for anything such as stress, anxiety, tension, pain, depression, exhaustion. When you can let go of how you think the poses look and go into the feeling by closing your eyes it will feel like a coming home. Inside you is not only love but spirit and it longs to nurture you, your hands can be the massages you need. Your body is your best friend; use these poses as a sacred connection between you and your body. I will give you the instructions although you add the fun sacred play. Think back to when you were a child, how you loved to be a explorer with your body. Let's learn from when we were kids and it was natural to use the body for play.

The most important part of this body relating is taking time and leave a full minute of lying down and tuning into peace and quietness at the end of each practice session. The obvious benefits of doing this is to feel the relaxation in the mind, body and emotions. Although healing of the body also come into account because if you jump up and get on with your day immediately after yoga the tight places stay in the same created pattern in the body. It is with total relaxation that the new pattern of lightness can be created.

Also just with the law of Attraction we can build a strong intuition and trust by spending a few moments in gratitude for your inner wisdom at the end of your routine. The more you begin to listen to your body, the more you pay respect to it the stronger the advice will present it self to you.

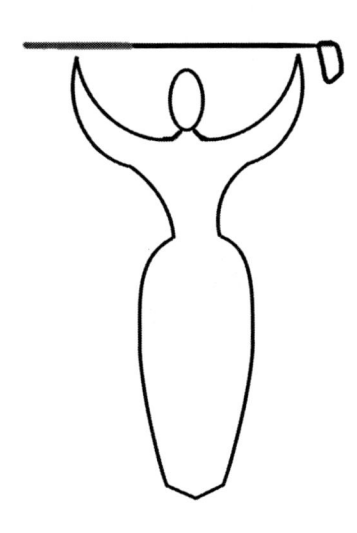

Fire

Physiologically Fire Poses increase body heat and energize the entire body.

I want to give special attention to the Sun Salutation. This is an Eastern ritual, a greeting to the sun every morning. It is not viewed as part of a fitness regimen like here in the Western Culture.

Because of our sedentary lives the phrase "what you don't use you lose" separates us not only from nature but from our Eastern family who do this daily. It is very natural for them to do this since the habit has become an unconscious act and is performed in an effortless way.

In the Yoga World the Sun Salutation is the perfect Whole body warm-up before doing any other yoga poses. Like the one-minute moon sequence it is a flow from one movement to the next. Inside this flowing routine are some very beneficial poses that can be and should be practiced all on their own. Now because I have worked a lot with Seniors and very stiff golfers I came up with a Golfers Sun Salutation that I will recommend starting with and not even as a warm-up before other poses. You could do one sitting of three like the one-minute moon sequence. However it does take longer to Master the breathing with the movements into a nice rhythmic flow, but the rewards are worth it. The full Sun Salutation instructions are not added to this beginner book, although you can easily find it on-line if you do wish to add it into your routine.

Leg Lifts and hold

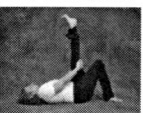

Warm-up before Golfers Sun Salutation –
Benefits- Releases tight Hamstrings, warm-up for legs, hips and low back
- Lie on your back, bend just your right knee and put right foot on the floor.
- Point the toes of extended left foot, inhale raise the leg.
- As you exhale, flex the foot and lower the leg.
- Repeat leg lifts four times: then hold the left leg with your hands inter locked on the back of the hamstring or leg, press leg into hands for 5 breaths. Change legs.

Preparing for Golfers Sun Salutation in which Sphinx replaces Cobra and Puppy Replaces Downward Dog.

Sphinx

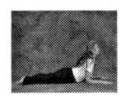

Gentle Back Bend a great Warm up for Cobra
- Lie flat on your belly, forehead on the floor, arms to your sides
- Bring legs together and point your toes back
- Inhale your head, chest and arms up and rest on your forearms
- Breathing your looking straight ahead or close your eyes.
- As you exhale, lower your torso first, then bring head slowly back to the floor.

Cobra

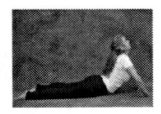

Benefits- Strengthens wrists, arms, shoulders, upper back and stomach muscles
- Lie flat on your belly, separate your legs to hip width and point your toes back
- Bend your elbows and place your palms on the floor in front of you with the fingers pointing towards each other.
- Put your forehead on the floor and relax your shoulders, as you inhale raise your head first then chest, when you feel your lower back engaging, press your hands down and arch your spine until your looking straight ahead.
- As you exhale, lower your torso, and then head slowly back to the floor.

Child

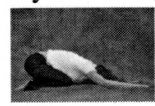

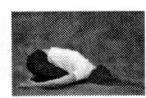

Benefits- A counter pose for any back bends, deeply calms and tranquilize the mind and emotions. This resting pose helps relieve low back pressure that happens when first beginning yoga.

Precaution- If knees are weak and feel too much pressure with the buttocks lowered to towards the feet. Place a cushion between at the back of the legs and sit down on it.

As an alternative to child begin with Puppy and work towards child, or reverse Child by laying on your back and hugging your knees into your chest.

Puppy

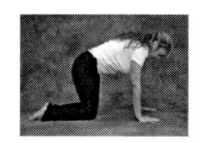

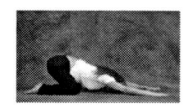

Benefits- stretches hips, lengthens shoulders, arms and back.
1. From a position of hands and knees
2. Stretch arms out in front and bring forehead to the floor.
3. Lean your hips back slightly, do not lower then towards the buttocks.

Downward Dog

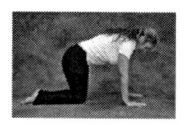

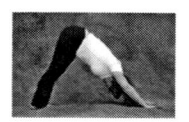

Benefits- Lengthens and stretches muscles, ligaments and nerves in backs of legs and spinal column. Opens shoulders and releases tension Nourishes facial skin, scalp, hair roots and enhances memory.
1. From a position of hands and knees, your fingers are spread apart on the ground pointing forwards.
2. Curl your toes under and press your hips into the air, straightening your legs. Then lower your heels as much as you can and bend the knees so you can aim your head back to touch them. This way the weight shifts back to your legs instead of your hands and wrists.
3. Your head is between your arms, and you are looking behind you through your legs, with practice your legs will straighten and the heels will be on the floor.
4. Try to hold for an extra breath, each time you do this so that your muscles lengthen.
5. To release, bend your knees and return to starting position.

Lunge with variations- stretches hips and hip flexors, back of legs

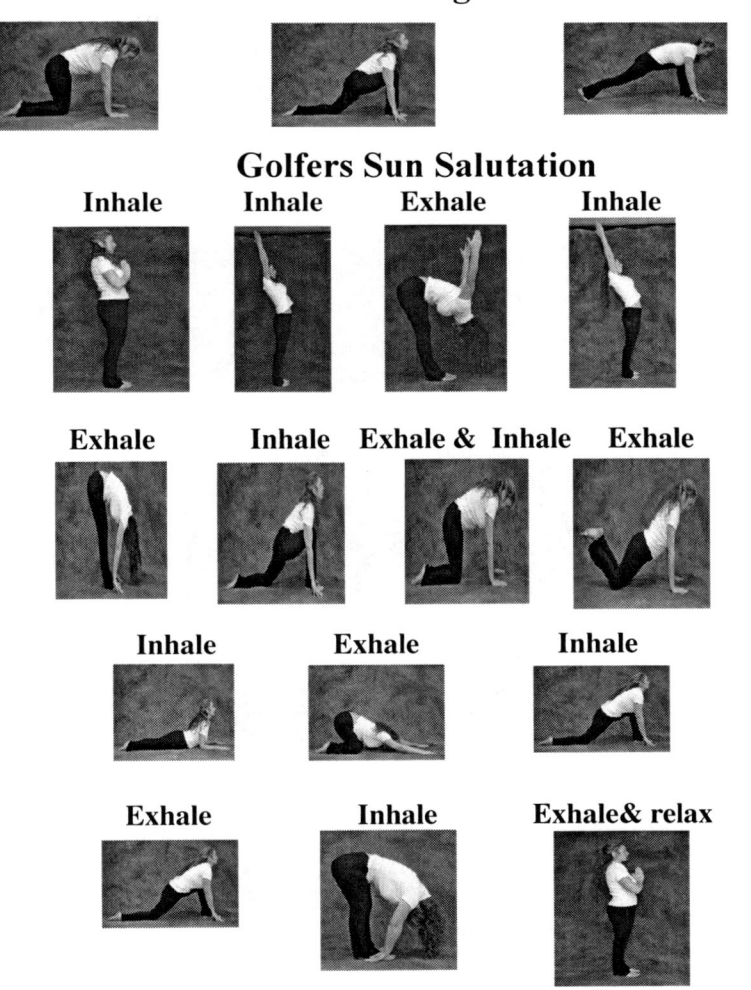

Golfers Sun Salutation

Inhale   Inhale   Exhale   Inhale

Exhale   Inhale   Exhale & Inhale   Exhale

Inhale   Exhale   Inhale

Exhale   Inhale   Exhale & relax

Repeat one more time for a full complete round.

Benefits- Provides an excellent warm-up sequence for stretching, toning and invigorating the whole body.

Improves muscle structure throughout the body: ankles, calves, knees, thighs, hips, abdomen, back, wrists, arms, shoulders and neck.

Come, Be Golfing Goddesses!

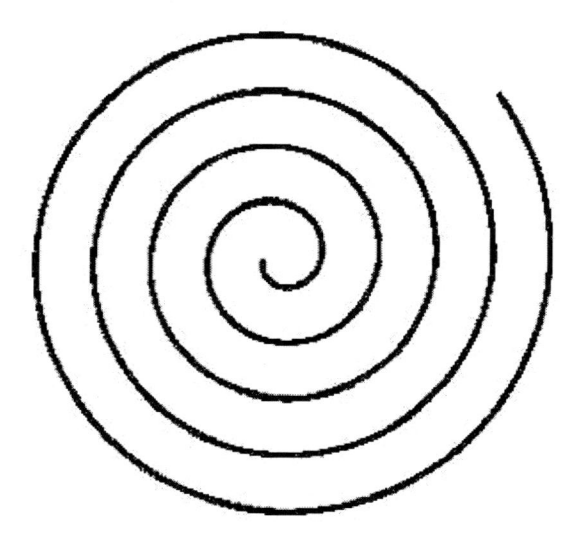

Triangle

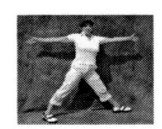

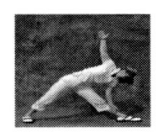

Benefits- Increases flexibility in the hips, ankles and knees, strengthens and stretches lateral, dorsal and intercostal muscles

1. Start in standing position, step legs apart four to five feet,
2. Inhale turn left foot out 90 degrees so it is pointing forward and right toe pointing inward 15 degrees.
3. Lift your arms out to the sides in a T position.
4. Lower right arm down to the right knee and extend the left arm overhead. Hold for a few breaths
5. Repeat on the other side.

Warrior 2

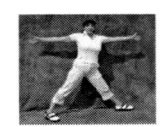

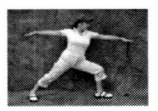

Benefits- Strengthens the feet, ankles, knees, thighs, hip joints. Strengthens and tones inner thigh muscles

1. Start with the legs in the same position as in Triangle
2. Inhale turn left foot out 90 degrees so it is pointing forward and right toe pointing inward 15 degrees
3. Exhale bend left leg so knee is over toes and turn head to the left. Breathe while hold 10 seconds and repeat on opposite side. Can be done with a club or without

Come, Be Golfing Goddesses!

Water

Physiologically Water poses develop qualities of receptiveness and sensitivity they can calm the mind and release emotions.

Frog

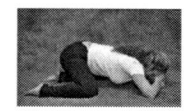

Benefits- Opens groin and hips
1. Start on your hands and knees, place your knees a little wide then hip width apart
2. As you exhale, sit back towards your heels, rest your torso on your thighs and your forehead resting on your hands which are placed in front of you. One hand on top of the other.
3. Breathe 4 to 6 breaths, if the stretch is easy open legs wider for a few more breaths.

Spinal Twist- easy   **advanced**

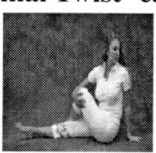

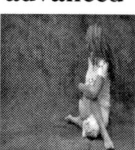

Benefits- Rotates and fully extends and aligns the spine, Removes stiffness from shoulders and neck.
1. Start from a sitting position with both legs extended out in front for easy twist.
2. Bend the left leg and cross the left foot over the right leg and place the foot flat on the floor on the outside of right knee.
3. Hold the knee with your right hand or and place your bent elbow on the outside of the left knee. –
4. Place the left hand behind your back, palm down on the ground and look over left shoulder
5. Hold the twist 6 to 8 breaths and repeat on the opposite side.

Bridge

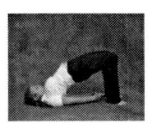

Benefits- Strengthens legs, buttocks & back, removes stiffness from shoulders
1. Lie on your back, knees bent, feet flat on the floor at hip width.
2. As you inhale, raise your hips to a comfortable height
3. As you exhale, return hips to the floor
4. Repeat steps 2 & 3 a few times, then hold the pose for 6 to 8 breaths
5. When holding shrug shoulders underneath and clasp hands together and press arms towards buttocks

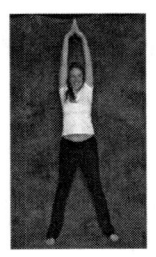

Half Moon

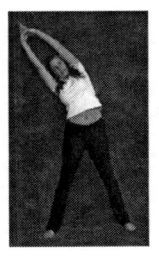

Benefits- Strengthens and tones every muscle in the central part of the body especially the obliques. Strengthens ankles, knees, hips, back, shoulders and neck.
1. Inhale arms over head, interlock hands to keep arms beside the ears.
2. Exhale bend to the side, check if breathing is short and tight if it is ease the bend up a bit until breathing is smooth hold for 10 seconds and switch sides

Standing Yoga Mudra

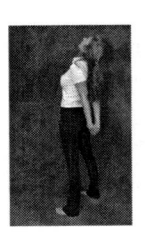

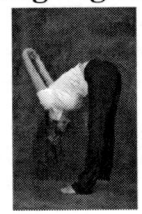

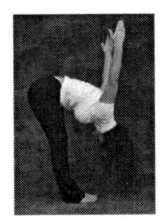

Benefits- Increases flexibility in arms, shoulders and spine and hips. Stretches muscles, ligaments and nerves in back of legs.
1. Bring hands together behind the back and clasp them together. Drop arms down and out behind for a breath or two.
2. Bring arms close to body while inhaling with the exhale bend forward with hands still clasped or unclasped if there is too much tightness.

Come, Be Golfing Goddesses!

Earth

Physiologically Earth poses promote strength, self-confidence and grounding. The balancing poses offer benefits of focus and concentration.

Extended Table

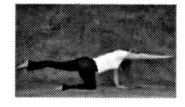

Benefits- Strengthens wrists and arms, balancing spine and strengthening torso.
1. Begin on your hands and knees, place your hands directly under your shoulders.
2. Lift your right arm and left leg off the floor in a comfortable position and hold for 4 to 6 breaths
3. Repeat with opposite pairs

Slow Motion Firming

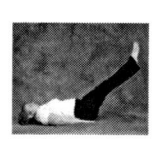

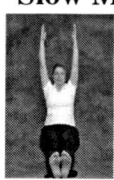

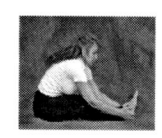

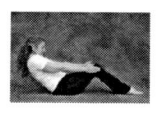

Benefits- Core Builder- Strengthens abdominals, low back, legs & buttocks a flow sequence for the core
1. Lie on your back, place hands underneath your buttocks. Inhale bend knees and then extend them to the sky in one breath.
2. Begin to exhale as you slowly lower your legs, continue to breathe, as you ever so slowly lower legs to the floor.
3. When your body is flat on the floor, inhale your arms over your head
4. With a strong exhale, pull your body up to a seated position and then bend over your legs
5. Hold the forward bend for 2 or 3 breaths
6. Bend your knees with feet flat on the floor, arms stretched out at the sides of your bent knees
7. Begin with an exhale and slowly roll back until you are flat on the floor once again.
8. Repeat steps in a slow continuous movement for a set of 3 to 5

Dynamic Knee Squeeze

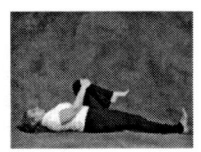

Benefits- Limbers Hips, releases low back pain, strengthens spine and neck.
1. Lie flat on your back, with both knees bent and feet on the floor.
2. Bend right leg and draw it into your chest, place hands on top or under neath knee.
3. Hold for 6 to 8 breaths
4. As you exhale, lift your head off the floor and hold for a breath or two.
   - Repeat on the other side.

Lying down half lotus

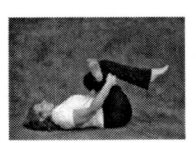

Benefits- Increases flexibility in the hips, groin, gluts, hip flexors & foot, stretches low back
1. Lie on your back, with both knees bent, feet flat on the floor.
2. Bring right ankle to top of left knee.
3. Inhale and raise left leg, on the exhale clasp hands either underneath or on top of left leg.
4. Keep left leg drawn into the chest and hold for 6 to 8 breaths.
5. Eventually bring the right foot down onto of the left thigh and hold for a couple of breaths.
6. Repeat on the other side.

Knee down Twist

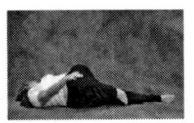

Benefits- Increases range of motion by fully rotating the spine, flexibility to spine, shoulders hips and neck.
1. Lie on your back, with both legs extended, arms out shoulder width, so you form a letter T
2. Place the bottom of your left foot on top of your extended right knee.
3. Inhale and bring your right hand on the outside of your left knee.
4. As you exhale, draw the left knee down to the right. Make sure the left shoulder stays on the ground.
5. Hold for 6 to 8 breaths, change sides.

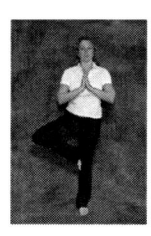

Tree Pose

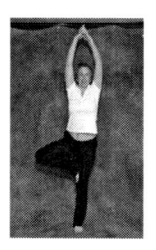

Benefits- Develops strong feet and legs, opens hips and lengthens spine, added benefit of concentration and focus.
1. To begin any balancing poses it helps to find a focal spot to look at be fore beginning.
2. Stare at an unmoving object at eye level
3. Shift your body weight to your left leg
4. Bring right leg up and place the foot on inside of left leg. Either before or after the knee but not directly on the knee area.
5. Make sure right knee is not pointing forward
6. Hands are together in front of chest, breathing deeply
7. When focused, raise arms overhead, continue holding for a few more breaths.
8. Slowly come down and change sides
9. If it is difficult to balance use the wall for support.

Chair

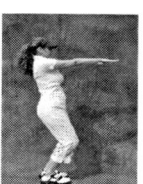

Benefits- Creates strong stable hips and legs, strengthens spine
1. From a standing position feet together
2. Inhale arms forward, shoulder height
3. Exhale bend knees, brings hips back as if preparing to sit
4. Press heels down and hold 20 seconds while breathing deeply

Standing Knee Squeeze

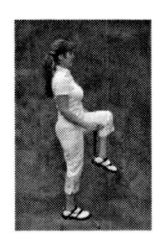

Benefits- Limbers hips, strengthens legs and spine, develops balance and coordination,
1. Standing tall keep your focus on an object in front of you
2. First practice without a club until you gain balance on both sides of the body.
3. On an inhale, raise bent knee up to your chest and either clasp hands on the outside of the bent knee or underneath it.
4. Hold the balance for a few breaths before changing sides
5. Do with and without holding onto a club

Dancer

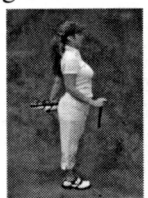

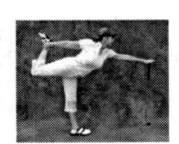

Benefits- Increases shoulder and spinal flexibility and strength, Tones abdomen, thighs, arms, hips, buttocks and legs
1. From standing position fix your eyes at a point in front of you.
2. Shift your weight onto your right leg. Bend the left knee and lift the left foot behind you towards your buttocks. Reach back and grab your left foot.
3. Hold this pose for a few breaths, then placing your right arm out in front of you lean forward into the stretch and hold here for a few breaths
4. Repeat on the other side, practice with and without a club

Forward Bend

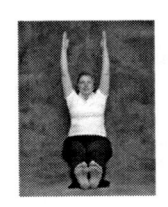

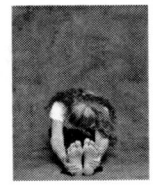

Benefits- Strength and flexibility of back and spinal column, stretches ham strings
1. Inhale arms overhead
2. Exhale bend forward from the hips, keep arms outstretched
3. Go as far as comfortable placing the hands on either, the knees, shins or feet. If hamstrings are really tight bend knees slightly
4. Hold the stretch, relax the neck and drop head and focus on breathing.
5. Coming out stretch arms out towards toes and bring them up over head with the inhale and exhale them down beside the body.

Head to Knee

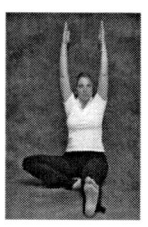

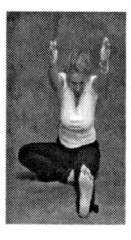

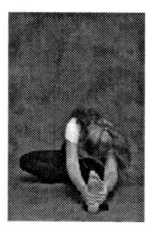

Benefits – and instructions are the same as the Forward Bend however with the knee bent into the opposite inner thigh it gives increased flexibility of the hips and opens the groins. It also relieves stiffness in the neck and upper back.

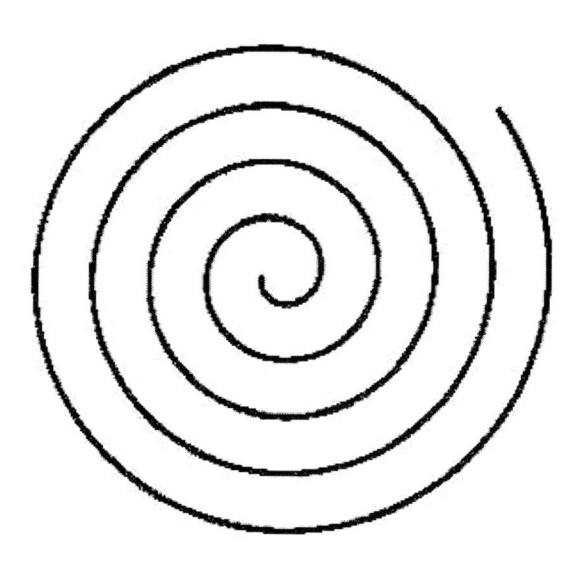

Air

Physiologically Air Poses represent freedom of Flight, they help build courage and release fear.

Rock the Baby

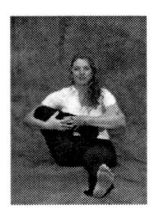

Benefits - Warm- up for Butterfly -targeting- hips and inner thighs
1. Sit on floor with legs stretched out in front.
2. Carefully lift your right foot up and cradle it in the crook of your left elbow, or hold in left hand.
3. Cradle your right knee in the crook of your right elbow.
4. Lift your spine and rock your right leg gently side to side 6 to 8 times
5. Shake out legs, repeat with left leg

Butterfly

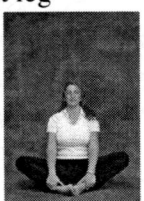

Benefits- Creates strong stable hips, stretches inner groin
1. Sit on floor and bring soles of feet together
2. Clasp either ankles or feet and draw feet in towards body
3. Hold the position for a few breaths, then begin to gentle bounce knees up and down, flapping your wings

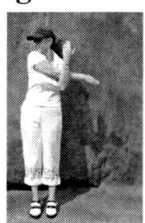

Eagle Warm-up | Beginner Eagle Pose

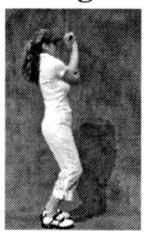

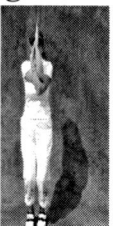

Benefits- Tones legs and upper arms, loosens and opens shoulders, develops focus
1. From standing position, bend knees and lower body as if sitting on a chair.
2. Draw arms out to the side and then cross them in front of you with the left arm on top of the right.
3. Bend the elbows and bring your forearms up toward your face. If possible clasp hands and interlace the fingers.
4. Breathe, it is easy to forget to breathe when you are in deep concentration
5. Hold for a few breaths, before repeating on the other side.

Half Locust

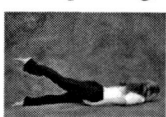

Benefits -Strengthens and tones legs, buttocks and low back and neck
1. Lie on your belly, with hands underneath your thighs, palms up.
2. With the chin on the floor, inhale and raise one leg up and away from the floor as high as comfortable for you. Press opposite leg into the floor.
3. Exhale lower the leg.
4. Repeat step 2 and 3 a few times, then hold the position for a few breaths.
5. Pause for moment before repeating with the opposite leg.

Beginner Pigeon

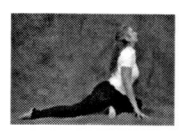

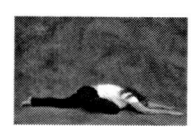

Benefits- World's best hip opener, tones back muscles
1. Start by coming onto your hands and knees.
2. Bend your left knee in front of your pelvis, lying it on the floor
3. Extend the right leg straight behind you along the floor and now the right heel should be underneath the right thigh.
4. Rest your fingertips alongside of left bent knee and press the torso in an

upright seated position.
5. If you are able, lower your head to the floor in front of you and take several deep breaths in this position. Repeat on other side.
6. Release this stretch by doing reversed Child, laying on your back and hugging knees into chest.

Specific Golf Fitness for Targeted Areas

"During an average 18-hole round, most recreational golfers take more than 100 swings. As well as walk six to eight kilometers and bend more than 30 to 40 times".
-David Lige

It's important to work these key areas of the body that are used in the golf swing. The benefit to the body and the game are as follows:

Legs and Hamstrings
strengthens ankles, quads and glutes
strong legs and hips support the body's ability to properly load & generate power and prevent the body from sliding

Hips
Solid foundation
Supports healthy back
Enables greater extension in the finish position of the swing

Core Strengthening/ Abdominals and back muscles
Essential for trunk rotation & power during the forward motion of the golf swing
Stabilizing factor throughout the golf swing

Back
Reduces risk of injury
Provides increased speed and power in the swing
Increases power and distance

Rotator Cuff
Common injury for golfers
Supports greater shoulder turn and club-head speed

Shoulders
improves shoulder turn in backswing
supports better posture at address and throughout the entire swing

Neck
Supports the body's ability to maintain proper head position during backswing

Hands & Wrists
Important as it's the only connection to the clubs

Yoga poses for targeted golf areas

Strength in the chest, shoulders, triceps and forearms is important for generating club head speed at impact.
- Sun Salutation
- Cobra
- Downward Dog
- Extended Table
- Half Cow & Cow
- Dancer

Well conditioned hamstrings help prevent lower back pain.
- Leg lifts
- Golfers Sun salutations
- Slow motion firming

Core exercises for abdominals help support and protect the lower back from injury, chronic area for golfers. Also these muscles are important in supporting the twisting and turning that occurs during the golf swing.
- Slow motion firming
- Cobra
- Half locust

Obloquies fire on the downswing, helping to accelerate your shoulders so that they catch up to your hips at impact. Strong obloquies help create speed

in your swing.
- 1 minute-Moon sequence
- Half moon
- Extended table
- Knee down twist
- Spinal twist

Strong legs are extremely important for anchoring the lower body. They support the rotation of your trunk and enable you to create more speed as you turn.
- Triangle
- Eagle
- Dancer
- Standing knee squeeze
- Sun salutation
- 1 minute-Moon sequence

Margarit Brigham © Copyright 2008

Bibliography

Steven Pressfield - *The legend of Bagger Vance*. William Morrow and Company 1995
Barbara G. Walker - *The Woman's encyclopedia of Myths and secrets*. Harper and Row 1983
Eric Chaline - *The Book of Gods and Goddesses*. HarperCollins Publishers Inc.
Napoleon Hill- *Think and Grow Rich-Fawcett Crest Book*-Ballantine Books
Masaru Emote - *The Hidden Messages in Water- Beyond Words* Publishing, Inc.

Come, Be Golfing Goddesses!

Resources – Books

Golf

Michael Murphy	GOLF IN THE KINGDOM
Steven Pressfield	THE LEGEND OF BAGGER VANCE
M. Scott Peck	GOLF AND THE SPIRIT
Tim Gallwey	THE INNER GAME OF GOLF
Pete Shoemaker	EXTRAORDINARY GOLF The Art of the Possible Fred Shoemaker
Dr. Bob Rotella/ Bob Cullen	GOLF IS NOT A GAME OF PERFECT
Dr. Bob Rotella/ Bob Cullen	GOLF IS A GAME OF CONFIDENCE
Pia Nilsson/ Lynn Marriott	EVERY SHOT MUST HAVE A PURPOSE
Debbie Steinbach Keller	VENUS ON THE FAIRWAY
Katherine Roberts	YOGA FOR GOLFERS

Goddess and Supportive Books

Barbara G. Walker	The Women's Dictionary of Symbols and Sacred Objects
Shinoda Bolen M.D	Goddesses in Every Woman Jean
Carol Bridges	The Medicine Woman Inner Guidebook
Nancy Blair	Amulets of the Goddess
Barbara Ardinger, Ph.D.	Goddess Meditations
Starhawk	The Spiral Dance
Louise L. Hay	You can heal your life
Estes Pinkola, Clarissa	Women who Run with the Wolves.
Caroline M. Myss	Anatomy of the Spirit
Marianne Williamson	A Woman's Worth
Doreen Virtue, Ph.D	Archangels and ascended Masters and Goddess Cards
Chungliang Al Huang/ Jerry Lynch	Thinking Body, Dancing Mind: Taosports
Wayne Dyer	Change your Thinking, Change your Life
Larry Dossey M.D.	Healing Words
Masaru Emoto	The Hidden Messages in Water
Echart Tolle	The Power of Now
Jamie Sams/ David Carson	Medicine Cards
Ted Andrews	Animal Speak
Dave Courchene Jr.	The Seven Grandfather Teachings
Dr. Seuss	Oh, the Places You'll Go

Resources

Websites
www.vision54.com
www.venusgolf.com
www.spiralgoddesses.com
www.yogajournal.com
www.theturtleloge.com
www.the8thfire.org
www.heartoftheintitiate.com
www.drumcafe.com
www.expertauthorpublishing.com

Favorite Charity's
www.golfandtheenviroment.org
www.adubondinternational.org
www.theturtlelodge.com

Margarit's Blogs
http://apps.yogaforgolf.ca/blog/ -tips for all golfers
http://golfgoddess.wordpress.com – female golfers
http://sacredconnections.wordpress.com – dedicated to Dave Courchene Jr.

Women's Golf Associations
Ladies Professional Golf Association LPGA-www.lpga.com Executive Women's Golf Association- www.ewga.com Royal Canadian Golf Association –www.rcga.org
Links for Women-www.linksforwomengolf.com
Golf fore Gals (B.C.)- www.golfforegals.com

Golf Equipment
Sandra Post -www.jazzgolf.com/sandra_post.php

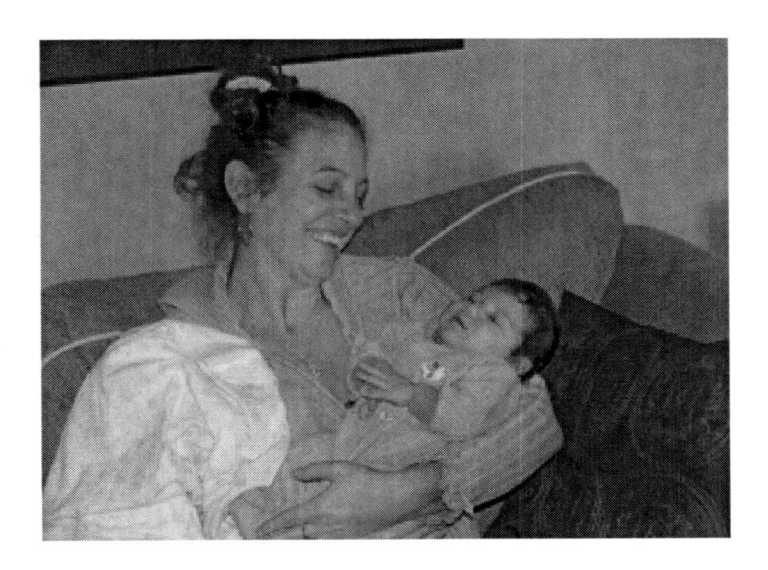

About the Author

Margarit Brigham who was given the nickname Peggy in her youth is a nature and an animal lover, and always takes the road less traveled in life and while walking in nature. She is a mother of two, a mother-in-law, and a Grandmother. She not only loves playing golf upon Mother Earth but also enjoys making crafts from the materials of the Earth. Margarit became a certified yoga teacher in 1995 and has continued her studies in yoga, spirituality, as a certified coach and Reiki Healer. She worked at golf courses for three years before becoming an entrepreneur in 1997 with Yoga for Golf. She was the sole owner and operated a yoga studio called 'The Yoga Connection' in Orangeville, Ontario for three years. Along with teaching her unique yoga programs she also developed and taught a 200-hour Yoga Teacher Training course, certifying 12 teachers. She is a professional speaker, workshop and retreat facilitator, freelance writer and her unique Yoga for Golf program was offered at the Toronto Yoga Show in 2006 and through the Learning Annex in Toronto. YFG has been featured in golf magazines, newspapers, and on Rogers T.V. Her newest project is fundraising and becoming a messenger and event coordinator for her favorite charity and teacher, Dave Courchene Jr. of The Turtle Lodge. Currently Margarit and her life partner Paulo live and play in North Vancouver, British Columbia.

For more information please visit her websites:
www.golfinggoddesses.com and www.yogaforgolf.ca